Forgiveness
The Healing Gift
We Give Ourselves

**THE PASSAGE TO
INNER PEACE
THROUGH
FORGIVING OTHERS**

Cheryl Carson

To my family members,
who were
my best teachers

COVER DESIGN AND LAYOUT: Sherrie Everett
COVER PHOTO: J. Blane Robinson

First Printing 1995

Sixth Printing
Revised and Expanded
1996

Table of Contents

Introduction

LEARNING TO FORGIVE was the greatest and most pain-filled struggle of my life. "There must be some kinda trick to this!" I thought in despair. "If I ever get it figured out, I'm going to share what I've learned with others who might be having a difficult time, as well."

I searched and studied, plead, wept, and prayed. When the breakthrough finally came, the burden lifted and the pain was gone. Perhaps others will benefit from knowing of the new ways of thinking, the new perspectives gained in my own journey.

As a frequent guest on the talk show of a radio station, I shared these insights regarding forgiveness with the listening audience on many different programs over the course of a year. The response was amazing; it seemed to have struck a chord in many people's lives.

After the first show, requests for copies of the material were so numerous that my husband and I decided to gather all the information I had shared—or intended to share—and compile it into a booklet. After four printings, it had expanded and become a 90-page book.

Once the project was conceived, it seemed to take on a life all its own. I felt as though I were being swept along in the current of a river to a predetermined destination. And, like the ripples that spread from dropping a pebble into a pond, the book has traveled far and wide.

This sixth printing contains four times as much material as the original booklet and includes insights and experiences that people have shared with me since the series on the radio began. It gives me great joy to offer this collection of the wisdom of so many. May your life be enriched, as mine has been.

The proverb states, "When the student is ready, the teacher will appear." The very fact that you have somehow come into possession of this book may indicate that you are now ready, that it is time for you to heal and to move on with your life. Perhaps you have suffered long enough.

May you begin to celebrate the light, the peace, and the joy that come when one has learned to forgive.

CHAPTER ONE

Resentment and Revenge

*He who pursues revenge
should dig two graves.*

—CHINESE PROVERB

A FTER READING THE original edition of this book, one woman wrote: "It answers many questions that seemed so unanswerable. Things I have learned internally after years of struggling but had not had verbalized before." Then she added, "For me, forgiveness came with difficulty, because I believed it was acquiescence—giving in. Such funny logic when it destroys you not to forgive. . . ."

I will not begin by quoting all the scriptures relating to forgiveness. If you have struggled with it as I have, you probably have them memorized. Besides, while I found them to say a great deal about the *requirement* to forgive, they did not seem to satisfy my need to understand *why* or *how*. It has been the greatest struggle of my life, this forgiving, even as I felt discouraged at my seeming inability to do so.

I believed that when one was wronged, feelings of anger would surely be justified. Wouldn't I have a right to feel angry? How can it be wrong to feel hurt if I *have* been hurt?

Of course, it would be easy to forgive someone who, upon recognizing his folly, came and begged my forgiveness. I would then be overcome with my righteous generosity and extend my forgiveness and good wishes to him. But what if that person who has wronged me never comes to beg? What if the offenses continue or if he never acknowledges his wrongdoing? Would it not be appropriate to want justice? If I forgive him for the dreadful things he has done and not paid for, then he would get off scot-free, and that would offend my sense of justice. How can I afford to back down by forgiving? Wouldn't that be admitting that he was right and I was wrong?

How to forgive, I don't know.
How can I let this anger go?
How many times be still and turn away?
Here with these hands I want to fight.
Here in my mind I want what is right.
Here on my knees I hold my heart and say,

"Take from me now all my bitter blaming.
Lift from my soul now the sin that's shaming me.
Give me, Lord, a love that's more than mine.
Bless me this day to cease demanding.
Let this poor heart now more understanding be.
Oh, give me, Lord, a heart like thine.

Help me to see with eyes more pure.
Help me to speak with lips of love.
Though I am wronged, find strength to rise above.

Help me to put my burden down.
Lighten my soul and let me live.
Grant me the gift to say, 'I will forgive.'
 —CAROL LYNN PEARSON, "I Forgive"

I felt somewhat confused — perhaps even offended — when I read the scripture which states, ". . . he that forgiveth not his brother his trespasses standeth condemned before the Lord; for there remaineth in him the greater sin" (D&C 64:9). I had a difficult time believing that if someone committed a major sin against me — betrayed or robbed me of something or someone precious to me — that it would be an even greater sin for me not to forgive him.

But then I realized that "sin" can be defined as anything that separates me from God or stops me in my own growth and progress — and, using that definition, my own feelings of lingering anger, bitterness, and revenge would be, for *me* the greater sin — simply because of what it did to *me*, ". . . *for there remaineth in him the greater sin.*"

Forgive: to pardon; to cease to bear resentment against; to cancel, as a debt.

Why does the Lord command us to forgive? For the same reason He gives us any commandment: for our own blessing and happiness and peace, now and forever.

3

Resentment—the Poisonous Emotion

Resentment, the opposite of forgiveness, has been called the "poisonous emotion." It has even been said that 80% of illnesses come from unresolved resentments. Indeed, I had heard of professional medical people who work with their patients by helping them to forgive. In his tape dealing with self-healing, one doctor said that, in order for self-healing to be effective, "you must be free of anger, loss of temper, holding grudges, resentments, ridicule, criticizing, condemning, finding fault, and casting blame."

Marion D. Hanks asked: "What is our response when we are offended, misunderstood, unfairly or unkindly treated, or sinned against, made an offender for a word, falsely accused, passed over, hurt by those we love, our offerings rejected? Do we resent, become bitter, hold a grudge? Or do we resolve the problem if we can, forgive, and rid ourselves of the burden? The nature of our response to such situations may well determine the nature and quality of our lives, here and eternally.

". . . Not only our eternal salvation depends upon our willingness and capacity to forgive wrongs committed against us. Our joy and satisfaction in this life, and our true freedom, depend upon our doing so. When Christ bade us turn the other cheek, walk the second mile, give our cloak to him who takes our coat, was it...out of consideration for the bully, the brute, the thief? Or was it to relieve the one aggrieved of the destructive burden that resentment and anger lay upon us?

"Even if it appears that another may be deserving of our

resentment or hatred, none of us can afford to pay the price of resenting or hating, because of what it does to us. If we have felt the gnawing, mordant [corrosive, as an acid] inroads of these emotions, we know the harm we suffer" ("Forgiveness, the Ultimate Form of Love" *Ensign,* Nov. 1973).

Pass Quickly Through Them

Voltaire observed: "Life is thickly sown with thorns and I know no other remedy than to pass quickly through them. The longer we dwell on our misfortunes the greater is their power to harm us."

One woman acknowledged the futility of harboring resentments toward those who have hurt her when she stated simply, "I refuse to rent out space in my brain to them." She explained, "There is only so much room in my mind, and I choose to fill it instead with thoughts of people I love. I won't rent out space to them." While not overflowing with compassion perhaps, her comment did demonstrate her common sense approach to emotional health.

Nurturing Grievances

I have met people who could recite long lists of grievances and hurts collected throughout their lives. None of them has seemed very happy people, however. I've never known anyone able to harbor resentments or bitterness and still maintain an attitude of gratitude or a sense of serenity. They are mutually exclusive; resentment and peace cannot co-exist. When one chooses to dwell on the pain of his injuries, he has, at the same time, chosen to turn his back on the joy of his blessings.

After being bitten by a rattlesnake, one can either, through fear or anger, pursue the creature with the intent to kill it—or he can turn his attention from the snake and concentrate his efforts on removing the venom from his own body as quickly as possible. One course could mean death to the rattler *and* the one bitten; the other is more likely to result in their mutual survival.

Harry Fosdick observed, "Hating people is like burning down your own house to get rid of a rat."

I read of one woman who kept a "hate book." Every time her husband did something to annoy or offend her, she wrote it down in her book, saying silently, "Another nail in your coffin." If one looks for nails, they can be found. Embittered people can usually explain in great detail the reasons for their resentments. They have tangible evidence in the nails they've collected. Ultimately, however, they are nails in their own coffins.

Frederick Buechner offers this graphic description: "Of the seven deadly sins, anger is possibly the most fun. To lick your wounds, to smack your lips over grievances long past, to roll over your tongue the prospect of bitter confrontations still to come, to savor to the last toothsome morsel both the pain you are given and the pain you are giving back—in many ways it is a feast fit for a king. The chief drawback is that what you are wolfing down is yourself. The skeleton at the feast is you."

"An Eye for an Eye . . ."

I once heard of a man who was offended by the water master. He said angrily, "I will never use another drop of water as long as he is the water master." Interesting logic. And thus we waste our lives trying to even up the score.

Forgiveness, on the other hand, has been defined as a creative violation of all the rules of keeping score. It is surrendering my right to hurt you back.

Surely we can see that nurturing resentments and seeking revenge are not in our own best interest. They are self-defeating. It is wise counsel to "be patient in afflictions, revile not against those that revile. Govern your house in meekness, and be steadfast" (D&C 31:9).

Resentment is the desire for revenge lying in wait. To seek revenge only perpetuates the transgression—this time, by *us.* Without forgiveness, injury begets injury, hurt for hurt, until revenge has run its course in mutual destruction. As Gandhi said, "An eye for an eye for an eye for an eye, and pretty soon everybody is blind."

Ah, "sweet revenge," the saying goes. A contradiction of terms, I believe. For, as the Count of Monte Cristo learned too late, revenge is not sweet but bitter indeed. He who has pursued it finds that, rather than feeling satisfied, he has given up his chance for life and love.

Clearly, resentment and revenge are obstacles to our own health and happiness. Harboring such feelings destroys our peace and blocks the flow of love in our lives. Perhaps there is a better way. . . .

CHAPTER TWO

An Act of Self-Love

*Forgiveness is an act of self-love
rather than simply an
altruistic, saintly thing to do.*

DANNION BRINKLEY DIED after being struck by lightening. He revived and later recorded his experience: "After the life review was over, the Being of Light gave me the opportunity to forgive everyone who had ever crossed me. That meant that I was able to shake the hatred that I had built up against many people. I didn't want to forgive many of these people because I felt that the things they had done to me were unforgivable. They had hurt me in business and in my personal life and made me feel nothing for them but anger and disdain.

"But the Being of Light told me I had to forgive them. If I didn't, he let me know, I would be stuck at the spiritual level that I now occupied.

"What else could I do? Next to spiritual advancement, these earthly trespasses seemed trivial. Forgiveness flooded my heart, along with a strong sense of humility. It was only then that we began to move upward" (Dannion Brinkley, *Saved by the Light*, 159–160).

Earlier in my life, I had never been aware that forgiveness was even an issue for me. The only time I remember consciously dealing with it was as a nineteen-year-old in college. I dated a charismatic but indecisive graduate student whom I adored pathetically. He took me on an emotional roller coaster ride through an entire semester. After a summer of corresponding occasionally, I returned to college in the fall, expecting to resume the relationship. Instead, I was stunned to learn that he was being married the next day to someone else. My feelings were a mixture of shock, pain—and even relief.

I remember sitting in church services a short time later, the words to the hymn sinking deep into my soul: *Fill our hearts with sweet forgiving; Teach us tolerance and love.* Suddenly I realized that I would not progress or go forward in my own life until I had forgiven him—and it was done. Later in my life, how I wished forgiveness could have been so easy.

To forgive a man costs me nothing. Suppose he has defrauded me, injured my reputation, attempted my life. What would I gain by refusing to forgive him? To reduce him to poverty would make me no richer. To destroy his peace would not heal me. To ruin his reputation would restore no luster to my name. To take his life would not lengthen my own life by a single hour.

Loss or Gain?

Perhaps only one obstacle prevents us from forgiving others. It is the belief that we are not the one who receives the benefit of our forgiveness. Unconsciously, we may associate forgiveness with loss instead of gain. Yet, consider, who carries the burden of the painful memories of the hurt? Who is consumed by negative thoughts, affecting other relationships? Who feels unworthy and isolated from God? Is it not the unforgiving one? Why do we believe that to forgive another would result in our loss?

To release ourselves from hard feelings of bitterness, hatred and unworthiness; to open our hearts to the flow of love and joy; to enable ourselves to heal—these are ways that forgiving others benefits us. Forgiveness is the path to our own freedom and peace. Forgiveness is for our own growth and progress.

To Hate or to Love

Psychiatrist George Ritchie, author of *Return from Tomorrow*, tells this story of "Wild Bill" (named for his mustache), one of the death camp survivors with whom Ritchie worked after the liberation:

"Wild Bill was one of the inmates of the concentration camp, but obviously he hadn't been there long: His posture was erect, his eyes bright, his energy indefatigable. Since he was fluent in English, French, German, and Russian, as well as Polish, he became a kind of unofficial camp translator. . . .

"Though Wild Bill worked fifteen and sixteen hours a day, he showed no signs of weariness. While the rest of us were drooping with fatigue, he seemed to gain strength. . . .

"I was astonished to learn when Wild Bill's own papers

came before us one day, that he had been in Wuppertal since 1939! For six years he had lived on the same starvation diet, slept in the same airless and disease-ridden barracks as everyone else, but without the least physical or mental deterioration. . . .

"Wild Bill was our greatest asset, reasoning with the different groups, counseling forgiveness. 'It's not easy for some of them to forgive,' I commented to him one day, . . . 'So many of them have lost members of their families.'

"'We lived in the Jewish section of Warsaw,' he began slowly, the first words I had heard him speak about himself, 'my wife, our two daughters, and our three little boys. When the Germans reached our street they lined everyone against a wall and opened up with machine guns. I begged to be allowed to die with my family, but because I spoke German they put me in a work group.'

"'I had to decide right then,' he continued, 'whether to let myself hate the soldiers who had done this. It was an easy decision, really. I was a lawyer. In my practice I had seen too often what hate could do to people's minds and bodies. Hate had just killed the six people who mattered most to me in the world. I decided then that I would spend the rest of my life — whether it was a few days or many years — loving every person I came in contact with.' This was the power that had kept a man well in the face of every privation."

Forgiveness Heals

Forgiveness is truly an act of self-love, the healing gift we give ourselves. To hate is easy — it takes no moral strength — but it is healthier to love. Forgiveness is the pathway to love, and love is always the answer to healing of any sort. Blame keeps wounds open; forgiveness heals.

"When our grievance grows to hatred, we become slaves of the very persons we hate. We are bound to them with chains that leave us no peace. Waking, we are haunted by their presence. Our sleeping is shadowed by their deeds. Our memories are clouded by their wrongdoing. Their present actions grind and gore us. We have allowed hatred to become our incarceration" (Karen Burton Mains, 'The Key to a Loving Heart," *Guidepost Books*, 78).

One woman described her feelings as she was able to forgive: "I'll never forget that Tuesday morning in my kitchen when I actually experienced the miracle of forgiveness. The windows of heaven were open and so much joy, happiness and laughter filled my soul, I could not control them. I also felt my Heavenly Father's great love for me and His forgiveness for the things I had done wrong. What a cleansing. I actually felt squeaky clean.

"The misery we put ourselves through for not forgiving others is crazy when we could be gaining spiritual growth and happiness" (Ilene Condie, *Church News*).

Lavater agreed when he said, "He who has not forgiven an enemy has never yet tasted one of the most sublime enjoyments of life."

CHAPTER THREE

My Own Journey to Forgiveness

"Jesus Christ had died for this man;
was I going to ask for more?"

—CORRIE TEN BOOM

ALL OF US, I'm certain, are aware of the Lord's requirement to forgive. The scriptures are replete with admonitions to do so, such as: "I, the Lord, will forgive whom I will forgive, but of you it is *required* to forgive all men" (D&C 64:10, emphasis added).

As I searched the scriptures in my own lengthy struggle to forgive, I felt disappointed—dissatisfied that there seemed to be little help in teaching me *how* to do it.

As previously mentioned, I had had little experience in consciously dealing with forgiveness in my life. Even after my second divorce and the depression that had followed, when it was suggested to me that I needed to forgive people in my life, I had to have help thinking of who those people might be. Former husbands were suggested as a start. Parents were also mentioned.

Forgive my parents? For what? I considered myself blessed to be a part of a perfect family, as close-knit as they come. Family members had always been there for me, helping me to know how I should think and feel (sometimes I even took notes). I was so grateful that they cared; I felt so loved. In fact, when I had written a book on adversity, I had dedicated it "to my dearest family, without whose love and support I could not have traveled far."

But all that changed for me in a drastic way five years ago. Something dreadful happened that turned out to be one of the greatest blessings of my life—although sometimes I wish my blessings didn't come in such disguise! Ultimately, it brought about changes in my life for which I will be eternally grateful. But I'm getting ahead of my story.

I will share the account of my own journey, as experienced and perceived by me at the time.

Not believing that my five grown nieces and nephews could be telling the truth about the tragic abuses they reported suffering as children — and viewing my own lone support of them and participation in the investigation as a personal and dangerous attack upon the family — the members of my family of origin decided they should "pull the covered wagons into a tight circle" and cut me off from any further association with them.

While I recognized that they were motivated by fear, still those three years before I learned to forgive were the most painful of my life. My physical suffering and recovery from a craniotomy for a brain tumor that occurred at the same time, was nothing compared to the emotional anguish of being cut off from the family I had thought of as extremely loving and upon whom I had earlier depended for my own sense of self-worth and security.

To be excluded from every wedding and reception and every missionary going and coming of nieces and nephews I had loved since birth, was very painful to me. It hurt to be removed as editor of the monthly family newsletter I had begun several years before, invited to cease contributing to it, as I would no longer be receiving a copy. Even my birthday was no longer acknowledged in the list of birthdays included in it.

And each time I received a letter from a family member, I was thrown into an emotional tailspin from which it took days or weeks to recover. Still, I kept those letters in a special file, tangible evidence of their cruelty to me and of my own righteousness in not responding to them.

Yet, I felt no peace. The turmoil within me was all-consuming. A wise friend observed: "You are building a museum to your pain." She suggested that I, figuratively, clean out that museum and fill it instead with the light and love of the Savior. "Look around you," she said. "They can't hurt you physically. You are surrounded by everything you need for happiness." That evening I burned the letters I had been saving.

I had been blessed to meet and marry a most wonderful, devoted, and supportive man, experiencing an unconditional love and acceptance that I had never known before. And although I had never been able to bear children in my previous marriages, shortly after the craniotomy and at exactly the same time as my disfellowshipment from my family became official, I conceived my first "homemade" baby and, at the age of forty-one, gave birth to a beautiful, healthy daughter, Merrie Anne. She has been a constant, tangible reminder of Heavenly Father's love for me and of His mindfulness of my other losses.

I had hoped that the birth of this long-awaited miracle baby would serve as a catalyst for the healing of relationships. We sent out announcements of her birth to all family members, accompanied by invitations to her blessing and dinner afterward to those who lived within traveling distance. Not only were the invitations rejected by all, but one brother who had been designated as the family spokesman sent instead a six-page letter of explanation in which I was compared to a rattlesnake and referred to as a "disciple of Lucifer."

A civil war continued to rage inside me. I had felt totally justified in my wounded feelings, but I had to acknowledge also that my own heart was not right. My feelings toward my family were hard feelings of bitterness. I instructed Micheal, my husband, that if I should die, he was not to inform my siblings of my demise. If they didn't want to see me alive, I certainly didn't want to give them the satisfaction of seeing me dead! While intellectually I was very aware of the need to forgive—if only for my own good—still I struggled, unable to find such feelings in my heart. For over three years I struggled.

Ask for God's Gift of Forgiveness

I read the story of Corrie ten Boom and prayed repeatedly that I, too, would receive an instantaneous gift of forgiveness in my heart, as she had done.

Corrie ten Boom, a native of Holland, along with her sister, had been arrested and sent to a concentration camp because they had hidden Jews in their home during the holocaust. Through severe privations, Corrie survived. Her book, *The Hiding Place*, recounts the story.

After a speech in which she had preached about the love of God and His forgiveness, Corrie was approached by and recognized a man who had been one of the concentration camp jailers who had treated them in such a humiliating way. "His hand was thrust out to shake mine. And I, who had preached so often . . . the need to forgive, kept my hand at my side. Even as the angry, vengeful thoughts boiled through me, I saw the sin of them. Jesus Christ had died for this man; was I going to ask for more? 'Lord Jesus,' I prayed, 'forgive me and help me to forgive him.'

"I tried to smile, I struggled to raise my hand. I could not. I felt nothing, not the slightest spark of warmth or charity. And so again I breathed a silent prayer. 'Jesus, I cannot forgive him. Give me your forgiveness.'

"As I took his hand, the most incredible thing happened. From my shoulder along my arm and through my hand a current seemed to pass from me to him, while into my heart sprang a love for this stranger that almost overwhelmed me.

"And so I discovered that it is not on our forgiveness any more than on our goodness that the world's healing hinges, but on His. When He tells us to love our enemies, He gives, along with the command, the love itself" (*The Hiding Place*, 239).

But the prayed-for miracle did not occur in my own situation, despite my pleading. Even as I prayed for the miracle of forgiveness, I clung to the hurts of the ongoing offenses. I considered myself a victim, cruelly dealt with, unfairly accused. I was obsessed by the pain.

Focus on Their Good Qualities

I went to others for counsel and help. My friend told me of an experience she had years before when she had been hurt by the knowledge that her roommates had criticized and mocked her when she was out of their presence.

She decided that she would write a list of all the good qualities of her roommates and leave the list lying in a conspicuous place so they would find it and thus be consumed by guilt and remorse for their treatment of her—her own brand of revenge.

Instead, she discovered that as she contemplated and wrote of the good things about her roommates, her own heart changed and she no longer felt the spirit of resentment, but the spirit of love and appreciation. So I tried that, too. It wasn't enough.

Feel Sorrow for Them

I telephoned the late Reed Bradford for counsel after he delivered an address on forgiveness on the radio. "Help me to learn how I can forgive these people who are hurting me so badly, when the offenses are repeated and ongoing," I begged.

His kindly response: "Feel sorrow for them. They are depriving themselves of many great blessings." I recognized the truth in his words. I *wanted* to feel that love for them, but the pain I was harboring seemed so great.

Pray for Them

Matthew 5:44 says to "pray for them which despitefully use you, and persecute you." In church, I listened with rapt attention as a woman spoke of forgiveness and the power of prayer. She shared an example from her own life. She said, "Prayer is my best source for healing. It really works, and sometimes we get even more than we expect.

"We had just moved to a new town about 30 years ago. I had called a refrigerator repairman to fix our freezer. The way he handled his business and treated his customers upset me so much and caused so much resentment that I immediately sought the Lord in prayer to get those awful feelings removed. As I felt peace again, I prayed for the repairman that sometime he would have the gospel taught him so he could have the type of change in his heart to treat people in a fair way.

"About three months later, I saw him and his wife at our church services. Through inquiry, I learned that they had been baptized the week before. But the thing that really amazed me was that when I told the family of the new members, our oldest son said that he and another man had been the ones who had taught the family the gospel."

And so I prayed for my offenders. I prayed that *they* would change and become more Christlike. I even began to feel sorry for them—that they apparently were clueless as to the meaning of unconditional love in their own lives, since they were not able to offer it to others (namely, me)!

But if I didn't really *want* to let go and forgive, at least I *wanted* to want to.

My Own Relationship With the Lord

In a religion class I gained some important insights. Just as the experience between Joseph in Egypt and Potiphar's wife (in which he resisted her efforts to seduce him) was actually between Joseph and the Lord ("How then can I do this great wickedness and sin against God?")—I similarly realized that the situation with my family was not an issue between my family and me. It was really an issue between God and me. In the end, I would probably not be asked for a recounting of what others had done to me, but rather I would be asked for an accounting of the state of my own heart and if my relationship with the Savior had allowed me to love as He loved and to forgive as He forgave. My ability or inability to love and forgive was simply a reflection of my own relationship with the Lord.

Accept Christ's Offering

But it wasn't until later, when I was viewing a video depicting the last days and events of Christ's life, that the breakthrough finally came. Perhaps it was the music that reached the depths of my troubled soul, or perhaps my heart was finally prepared.

As I witnessed my Savior and what he was willing to suffer for me — as I watched the cruelty forced upon him, so undeserving of such treatment in his utter innocence and total purity — as I felt his love for me — my own heart overflowed with sorrow and love and gratitude for him. I began to weep openly. As the tears flowed, I felt as though my own heart was broken. My spirit was also contrite, and I felt ashamed.

I had been praying all along to be given the gift of the pure love of Christ and a forgiving heart. Now I realized that Christ had offered me that gift a long time ago. He had invited me to partake of his love and the healing power of his atonement, but until now I had simply not accepted his offering, his great gift. Until now, I had rejected his invitation to carry my burdens for me, to take upon himself my pain, and to allow me to partake of his peace.

I decided at that moment to accept his invitation, to let go of my pain and to turn the entire situation over to him.

> *As little children bring their broken toys*
> *with tears for us to mend,*
> *I brought my broken dreams to Christ*
> *because He was my friend.*
> *I snatched them back and said,*
> *"How can you be so slow?"*
> *"What could I do?" He said,*
> *"You never let them go."*
> —UNKNOWN

"The whole world lieth in sin, and groaneth under darkness . . . *because they come not unto me*" (D&C 84:49-50, emphasis added).

From that time on, after my heart-softening experience watching the video, I was able to turn it over to the Savior and obtain the peace and the freedom from constant pain that I so much had longed for . . . even as I yet had lessons to learn. From that time on, my heart was open to a new way of thinking, a new perspective. My mind was now open to new insights and new beliefs that would make forgiveness easy and painless—and would, ultimately, make it unnecessary.

CHAPTER FOUR

Taking Responsibility for Our Own Lives

*As long as we blame others
for the way we feel today,
we will have to wait for them to
change before we can be happy.*

—WAYNE DYER

FTER I EXPERIENCED the marvelous break-through in which I felt such a great love from and for the Savior and had surrendered my pain to Him—even after that—I continued to grow and to learn new things. Now concepts that I had heard or read before made real sense to me. Like the pieces of a puzzle, truths from many sources fell into place and fit together. They revolutionized my way of thinking about forgiveness, and I began to internalize principles that would eventually lift the burden of feeling forgiveness was something I *had* to do. Rather, practicing these principles removed the pain, and, eventually, forgiveness was no longer even an issue.

Taking Offense

It was an "Aha!" moment when I heard the concept regarding offenses. It was very simple yet life changing for me, as offenses had continued to come. It is this: In order for there to be an offense, a two-part transaction must take place. There must be one *giving* the offense and one *taking* offense. If the second party refuses to *take* offense—even when one is intended—the transaction cannot be completed.

From that moment on, I decided that I would simply choose not to take the offense when it was offered to me. What a wonderful, freeing feeling!

A simple analogy illustrates. Suppose I had grown up conditioned to believe that I must sample every kind of food offered me and that I must always eat everything on my plate. Imagine my being invited to a banquet at which a waiter offers me food that would be toxic to me.

Acting from my earlier conditioning and old beliefs, I might feel obligated to take and eat the food. But in learning to take responsibility for my own life, I realize that I need not eat anything unless I choose to.

Taking offense (whether intentional or not is irrelevant) is like ingesting a poison that would be harmful to my spiritual, emotional, and physical health. The offender may persist in offering, but I can decide whether or not to accept it. I can politely respond, "No, thank you," to the offense rather than taking a heaping helping of the hurt.

Brigham Young was credited as saying, "He who takes offense when none is intended is a fool. He who takes offense when it *is* intended is also a fool."

Taking Control of Our Lives

What a freeing feeling it is to realize that we can be in control of our own life. No longer do we need to feel like a helpless victim, acted upon by the cruelty or insensitivity or unfairness of others.

Indeed, we are responsible for all of our experiences. We fashion our future with every thought we think. Therefore, it is vital to our growth to forgive everyone. Holding onto past grievances only hurts us. The harm others have done to us in the past only matters to the extent that we allow it to affect us today.

The more we dwell on what we don't want, the more of it we create. Whether positive or negative, that which is focused upon will expand. Plants nurtured and watered will grow; those neglected will eventually wither and die.

God is love; therefore, love is permanent and all-powerful. Evil is temporary, without character of its own. Trouble has no life except that which we give it by nourishing it with our thoughts and emotional energy. Mentally going over old grievances, recalling the details, savoring the injustices, and cherishing the pain, revitalizes that which would have otherwise quietly withered and died of neglect.

The secret, as Christ taught, is to "resist not evil" (see Matt. 5:38-39). Wrestling with the injury fuels it with further life and power. Simply withdraw that thinking and emotion which give life to the difficulty. The harm exists only when it is fed and recharged by dwelling on it.

Ironically, the bitterness we may feel infects our whole lives while the other person is still on his or her path doing exactly what he or she knows how to do, regardless of our current miserable state.

No Need to Feel Threatened

When we take responsibility for our own lives and allow others to take responsibility for theirs, we will not feel threatened by their mistreatment of us. "What others think of me is really none of my business!"

Frederick Douglass was a man who fought for the advancement of colored people after the Civil War. "At one time Mr. Douglass was traveling in the state of Pennsylvania, and was forced, on account of his color, to ride in the baggage-car, in spite of the fact that he had paid the same price for his passage that the other passengers had paid. When some of the white passengers went into the baggage-car to console Mr. Douglass, and one of them said to him: 'I am sorry, Mr. Douglass, that you have been degraded in this manner,' Mr. Douglass straightened himself up on the box upon which he was sitting, and replied: 'They cannot degrade Frederick Douglass. The soul that is within me no man can degrade. I am not the one that is being degraded on account of this treatment, but those who are inflicting it upon me'" (Booker T. Washington, *Up from Slavery*, 100).

When we sense our divine worth, we need not feel threatened, because we are secure in that knowledge and in our relationship with the Lord. Only when we believe or fear that there is validity in another's mistreatment of us, will we feel a need to become defensive or to retaliate. Christ did not defend himself before Pilate; He knew who He was. Jesus went to Calvary in pain and agony; but Jesus went to Calvary in peace.

Forgiveness Is a Choice

We choose life for ourselves and others when we forgive. First, we relieve ourselves of the burden of carrying around hurt, anger, pain, isolation and darkness. Healing happens to us. Second, we give someone else freedom to live their life (or sometimes rest in peace) and work out their own feelings, behavior, and consequences. Thus, we are both allowed to take responsibility for our own lives.

Although we may have experienced pain, we don't need to remain victims, blaming those who have hurt us. If we do, we won't be able to forgive them. We want to see those who have hurt us as wounded children of God experiencing their own problems in mortality.

If we are having difficulty forgiving others whom we perceive as having wronged us, perhaps we would do well to examine our choice to blame them for our unhappiness. Perhaps our feelings of hurt and anger have progressed to hatred. This is *our* hatred. We carry it with us wherever we go. We own it; it is a burden we have elected to carry.

Unfortunately, we have given another person power and permission to not only hurt us once, at the time he did his dreadful deed, but to *continue* controlling our lives, blocking our passage to peace and happiness.

When we become aware that we can remove ourselves from the victim role, that we can choose to let go and forgive, we are actually freeing ourselves. It is as though we are saying, "I no longer give you control over my life. I will no longer allow you to affect how I will think and feel and act. I take responsibility for all of that now."

Spencer W. Kimball capsulized it: "In you alone is the control of your life — what you're going to be and what you're going to do. I hope that every one of you will make up your mind and say, 'I am going to be responsible for what I am, what I think, what I do, and [for] my life.'"

Wayne Dyer shares his personal insights: "I now know that I truly have no one to forgive, and I never did. I simply had to correct my misperception that others were causing me to be miserable, that they were the cause of my discontent. Paradoxically, through the act of forgiveness, I have come to the place where forgiveness never comes up for me. I have learned to accept others exactly as they are. . . . Consequently, acceptance has allowed me to see them for what they are and where they are, and to remind me of the same thing in myself. Any hostile or negative reaction in me, as a result of the behavior of others, really just lets me know where I am, or am not, and no longer requires any forgiveness. I have come to the point of not needing to forgive, by forgiving. One more paradox" (*You'll See It when You Believe It,* 264).

There's a story I like about two painters on their lunch break. One of them looks into his lunch box and protests, "Peanut butter again! I *hate* peanut butter!"

His fellow worker inquired, "Why don't you ask your wife to make you something else?"

"Oh, I'm not married," replied the first man. "I make my own lunches."

We, too, "make our own lunches." We may believe we are helpless—powerless in controlling the hurt we feel as a result of the actions of others. Not so! While negative, bitter thoughts may come to us uninvited, *we* decide whether or not we will entertain them. As someone said, "If *you* don't do your own negative thinking, nobody is going to do it for you."

We create our own lives, our futures, our happiness or misery by what we invite to occupy our minds and with what we choose to fill our hearts.

CHAPTER FIVE

"Judge Not"

*The greatest form of charity
is the withholding of judgment.*
—MARVIN J. ASHTON

THERE IS A seemingly magic formula that will make forgiveness easy—and, ultimately, make it unnecessary. It is found in the scriptures, although I had never before fully recognized the connection between it and forgiveness. It is so simple, it can be summarized in two words. It can be explained succinctly in a paragraph; and its benefits can be expounded upon at length. It is simply, "judge not."

You see, in order for me to feel there is someone I need to forgive, I would first have to judge that person as having wronged me. Even as I view myself as the victim, I am judging and accusing him of being a victimizer.

Surely it is desirable for us to evaluate and try to understand—and judging another with kindness and a generous heart cannot be wrong. But in the scriptural context, translated from the Greek, to "judge" means to "condemn."

Indeed, the admonition not to judge/condemn appears clearly in relation to forgiveness. Directly after the Lord instructed that we are to forgive all men, he said: "And ye ought to say in your hearts — *let God judge* between me and thee, and reward thee according to thy deeds" (D&C 64:11, emphasis added).

When I first encountered that scripture, I was in the midst of my struggle. It was palatable to me, satisfying my impure heart, as I interpreted it to mean that I needn't judge because God would be the one to punish those awful folks! Steven Cramer offered a more charitable explanation of the verse. "That may sound like a curse, but it is not. There is great healing when we let go of the pain, when we refuse to punish the offender, when we surrender the injustice to him who suffered the greatest injustice of all. Leaving the judgment of the offender to the Lord is the path to freedom and peace, even though the offense may not be righted" (*In the Arms of His Love*, 165–66).

One man related to me how he had decided that for a period of two weeks he would refrain from judging everyone. He described feelings of peace and joy in his experience. "It was like a tremendous burden had been lifted from my shoulders."

Another man shared a similar insight. "I have been guilty of judging—of trying to set right some wrong against me or others, as I perceived it. I then learned how much easier and more fulfilling life is when you let God do the judging. I learned that a big load is removed from my shoulders when I don't make it my responsibility to be judgmental. So much time and energy are wasted that could be spent on developing tolerance and love for others."

Deepak Chopra asserts that a vital contributor to health and well-being is to refrain from judging people or events. He urges us to avoid making any kind of assessment, appraisal, or evaluation, but simply to observe, without drawing conclusions.

Distress and "dis-ease" resulting from judging others are eliminated.

Nothing to Forgive

I began to realize that as I change the way I view life and other people, I no longer feel compelled to judge in a condemning way. There will no longer be a need to have to forgive, because there will be nothing to forgive. A rather traumatic experience I had some years ago illustrates this.

After church services one Sunday, my bishop called me into his office. Wishing to prepare me, he said kindly, "I just felt you should know that tomorrow you are being charged with child abuse."

My mind raced wildly, full of confusion. What had I done? The story came out. A few days earlier I had asked another mother in our neighborhood to care for our baby for the afternoon. When she changed the baby's diaper, she was alarmed to see numerous dark spots on the baby's lower back and buttocks. She called in her neighbor: "Do these look like birthmarks or bruises?" she asked.

Her husband happened to be a policeman, and she called him home. Unfortunately, neither he nor the five other policemen who joined him had ever heard of Mongolian spots.

Months before, we had adopted this baby from Korea. I had flown down to Los Angeles to meet the plane arriving with the babies and their escorts aboard. The first thing the escort had said to me was, "Now, don't be alarmed at what appear to be bruises on her lower back and buttocks. They are called Mongolian spots, and all dark-skinned babies have them. They will fade and disappear within a few years." I had thought nothing more of it.

Now, in the bishop's office, when the explanation for the misunderstanding dawned on me, my first reaction was to laugh. But then I cried—to think that all those people who knew me had thought me capable of inflicting such bruises upon my baby. It hurt.

When I got home, I called the bishop and read to him from the medical encyclopedia the description of Mongolian spots. He relayed the message and nothing more came of it.

I suppose I could have judged the woman who had noticed the spots—judged her to have meant me harm, set out to destroy my reputation, my family, my life, had my baby taken from me, sent me to prison, etc. But those kinds of thoughts never even crossed my mind. I knew that she had simply done what she was supposed to do: report a possible case of child abuse. How could I fault her for doing what she felt was right, even under difficult circumstances?

A few minutes after my telephone call to the bishop, the woman showed up on my doorstep, asking for my forgiveness. But there was nothing to forgive, because I had not judged her. We embraced and then sat on the steps together, sharing our feelings through the entire ordeal. When she had learned that the police were actually planning to press charges against me, she wanted to "back out" of her involvement, but it was too late. Nor would they allow her to speak to me about it. Actually, she had suffered far more than I, for she had been in agony for days, and my own pain had lasted only a relatively short time. Our friendship actually became stronger.

My own mother has been an example to me of judging my motives and the intent of my heart with kindness. Although she may disagree with what I have done, her message is, "I know that you felt you were doing the right thing."

God gives us the benefit of the doubt. In Psalm 78:37–39 we read: "For their heart was not right with him, neither were they steadfast in his covenant. But he, being full of compassion, forgave their iniquity, and destroyed them not; yea, many a time turned he his anger away, and did not stir up all his wrath. For he remembered that they were but flesh." (I can almost imagine Him saying of me, "She's only 45 years old; give her a break!")

If you are tempted to lose patience with your fellowmen, stop and think how patient God has been with you. Wendy Ulrich observed, "While we do not condone the sin, we do not condemn the sinner. We acknowledge the possibility that the Lord may, in his greater wisdom and knowledge of the full context of the sinner's life, have reason to be lenient. Trusting our own judgment of the wrongfulness of the *sin*, we nevertheless leave judgment of the *person* to the Lord. This blesses us with the assurance that the Lord will be merciful to us as well." (*Spiritual Recovery*, 355–56).

Judging Another's Heart

Oh, that men would see more clearly, or judge less harshly when they cannot see!

Marvin J. Ashton said, "If we could look into each other's hearts and understand the unique challenges each of us faces, I think we would treat each other much more gently, with more love, patience, tolerance, and care. Be one who nurtures and who builds. Be one who has an understanding and a forgiving heart, who looks for the best in people. . . ."

We must be slow to condemn and quick to forgive. We can recognize that those who may have offended us did what they knew how to do, given the conditions of their lives. One woman demonstrated her compassion when she said, "Many have not learned of God's love. How could they behave other than they do?" We're not put here on this earth to see through one another, but to see one another through.

I recall the account of a person traveling on the subway, annoyed by the obnoxious behavior of some young children. The father seemed lost in his own thoughts, seemingly ignoring the antics of the children.

"Can't that man control his own children?" thought the agitated traveler. "How rude of him to allow them to disturb other passengers like this!" She approached the man, suggesting that he restrain his offspring.

He turned to look at her, his eyes filled with pain. "I'm sorry," he said. "The children and I have just come from the hospital where we said goodbye to my wife and their mother for the last time."

How quick we are to judge others! Perhaps *we* should plead, "Father, forgive us, for so often we know not what we do."

Who am I to judge another when I walk imperfectly?
In the quiet heart is hidden sorrow that the eye can't see.
Who am I to judge another? Lord, I would follow thee.
—SUSAN EVANS MCCLOUD

It is utterly presumptuous of us to feel that we have the right to judge another's motives, the intent of his heart, to know all the events of his life that have influenced his way of thinking and behaving. If God "maketh his sun to rise on the evil and on the good, and sendeth rain on the just and on the unjust," then how can we mere mortals presume to have the right to judge and, based on that judgment, to decide who is and who is not deserving of our forgiveness?

In the movie, "Rudy," I was impressed when the Catholic Priest said, "There are two things I have learned in all my years: first, that there is a God; and second, that I'm not Him."

Someone else said: It is a great burden lifted to recognize "that we do not know the complete circumstances of the people who have had an impact on our lives. We do not possess the omniscience to be able to say, 'Dad should have been able to pay more attention to us kids,' or 'Mom shouldn't have been so uptight all the time.'

"Forgiveness acknowledges that we do not have the knowledge or the wisdom to sit as judge, jury, and executioner over people who have hurt us in the past."

We can acknowledge that each individual is responsible before God for his or her choices. We can rest assured that God is perfect in His knowledge, perfect in His justice, and perfect in His mercy—and thus the only one qualified to judge.

" . . . the Lord seeth not as man seeth: for man looketh on the outward appearance, but the Lord looketh on the heart" (I Sam. 16:7).

People Change

Another perspective that may be helpful in avoiding a condemning judgment of others is to realize that people change and grow. Looking back, there are many things I would have done differently in the situation with my family; I have learned and grown a great deal since then. I know of the pain that comes from being judged to be the same person I was years ago—an arbitrary and absolute judgment that negates the potential of God's children to progress.

The subject of people changing was addressed by one woman who wrote: "I read a quotation once that really impressed me. It said, 'I consider my tailor my best friend; he takes new measurements every time I see him.'

"If only we could all be like the tailor and realize that people change and grow. Too often we hold fast to our old measurements of people and fail to recognize they have changed for the better. How many of us when someone mentions the name, 'Scrooge,' think of the 'Bah, humbug!' miser at the beginning of Charles Dickens' story and not the repentant Scrooge at the end?"

Another woman shared this: "We should be able to look at others and realize they are new and larger souls because of their mistakes. None of us are the same individuals we were ten or even five years ago. Often, we wouldn't even recognize that person if it wasn't for physical characteristics and superficial mannerisms. Each of us is born anew each day.

"For instance, that person who hurt your feelings at church doesn't even exist anymore . . . We must kneel with broken hearts and ask the Lord to grant us the pure love of Christ that we may forgive and see each other through His eyes."

Judge with Compassion

It is not the event itself that determines our feelings, but our own assessment or judgment of the event that influences how it will affect us. Imagine being on an elevator. It stops and a man enters, stepping squarely on your foot. It is painful, and feelings of anger well up inside you.

Now, replay the exact same event. You are on the elevator. The man enters, squarely stepping on your foot. It is painful—only this time you notice that the man is carrying a white cane. Your feelings now may be entirely different from those of the first scenario. Rather than judging the man to have hurt you intentionally or out of negligence, you may look upon him with compassion, believing him to be doing the best he can, considering his handicap.

Steven Cramer expanded on this concept. "It is helpful to view those who repeatedly hurt us as being handicapped. Wouldn't it be easier to forgive them for hurting us if they were physically crippled or blind? Perhaps they are blind emotionally. Perhaps they can't see how they hurt others. Perhaps, because of unfortunate circumstances in their past, they just don't know any other way of relating to you. For all we know, their unacceptable behavior may be nothing more than a reflection of the way they were injured in their youth. If we could see into their hearts as God can, we would understand their deviant behavior and not condemn them for it" (*In the Arms of His Love*, 169).

"Why dost thou judge thy brother? Or why dost thou set at nought thy brother? For we shall all stand before the judgment seat of Christ. . . . Every one of us shall give account of himself to God. Let us not therefore judge one another any more; but judge this rather, that no man put a stumbling block or an occasion to fall in his brother's way" (Rom. 14:10, 12–13).

Wayne Dyer observed: "Judgment means to view the world as *you* are, rather than as *it* is. . . . When you judge another, you do not define that person, you define *yourself*.

"When you accept others, you no longer experience the hurt that goes with judging them. . . . If you do not judge those around you but instead accept them for precisely where they are on their own path, eliminating your need to be upset by them, you have put forgiveness into practice. Forgiveness is really just correcting our own misperceptions. You really have nothing to forgive, other than yourself for having judged or blamed in the first place" (*You'll See It When You Believe It*, 256–257).

CHAPTER SIX

All That We Give, We Give to Ourselves

*For that which ye do send out
shall return unto you again,
and be restored.*

—ALMA 41:15

I THOUGHT THAT I had covered the subject of forgiveness rather thoroughly in the six times I had been on the radio. But then came the phone call from a man named Don Clawson in which he added insights that had not even occurred to me. In fact, he pointed out some truths I had totally missed: the ultimate, *most* important reasons for forgiving others.

As he revealed them, I recognized the truths. Although I had heard these things all my life and all the scriptures he cited were already familiar to me, it was as though I had had an assortment of puzzle pieces that heretofore had been turned face down. Now I was finally turning them over, fitting them together, and seeing, for the first time, the completed picture of this vital concept of forgiveness.

These truths, simply stated, were: First, we will be forgiven of our own sins *only* if we are willing to forgive others of theirs.

Second, at the time of judgment, we will get back exactly what we gave. When we take the scriptures literally, it is very clear. We will be judged with the same measurement by which we have judged others.

The Demands of Justice

After the fall of Adam, our first parents and all their descendants were cut off from the presence of God. Justice would dictate that we remain forever in this lost and fallen state. But because God is merciful, a way was provided whereby an atonement could be made in our behalf. Because of Christ's love for us, He was willing to suffer for our sins, to pay that tremendous debt for us, in order to satisfy the demands of justice.

There are no requirements for Christ's love. His charity— which is defined as "the pure love of Christ"— is extended to sinners as well as saints. However, in order for us to receive the benefit of His atoning sacrifice, we must have faith enough to come unto Him and to repent of our sins. Repentance is simply the demonstration of our willingness to accept the Savior's invitation to turn from our sins and toward Him, to receive forgiveness, and to be able to dwell with Him and our Father again. And thus mercy can satisfy the demands of justice.

However, the Lord himself clearly states the final step of our repentance: "Wherefore, I say unto you, that ye ought to forgive one another, for he that forgiveth not his brother his trespasses standeth condemned before the Lord; *for there remaineth in him the greater sin*" (D&C 64:9, emphasis added).

The final step of our repentance and our being forgiven, then, is our willingness to forgive all others their trespasses against us. If we have followed all the steps of repentance to the end, and although we may have experienced recognition, remorse, made restitution, and resolved never to do it again—if we don't complete the final step, forgiving others, then it doesn't count! Our sins still remain with us and the atonement cannot take effect in our lives. As Catherine Marshall observed, "He who will not let us down also will not let us off. . . . The condition of having our sins cleansed is our forgiveness of others."

Furthermore, forgiving others is not merely an optional matter based upon our judgment of whether or not the other person has repented, is deserving, or has asked for our forgiveness. The continuing verse declares, ". . . of you it is *required* to forgive *all* men" (D&C 64:10, emphasis added).

Why We Should Forgive

A woman once telephoned me and related that she had earlier committed a serious sin and had felt that her relationship with God was in jeopardy. She desired with all her heart to receive His forgiveness, yet had recognized her unwillingness to forgive others. She told me then that it was as though the Lord was saying to her, "Wait a minute. You expect me to forgive you of this major transgression—yet you are not willing to do the same for others?"

Christ told a parable that illustrates this perfectly.

Interestingly, the caption in the chapter heading reads, *Why we should forgive.*

"Therefore is the kingdom of heaven likened unto a certain king, which would take account of his servants. And when he had begun to reckon, one was brought unto him, which owed him ten thousand talents [which, I'm told, is roughly $20,000,000!]. But forasmuch as he had not to pay, his lord commanded him to be sold, and his wife, and children, and all that he had, and payment to be made. The servant therefore fell down, and worshiped him, saying, Lord, have patience with me, and I will pay thee all. Then the lord of that servant was moved with compassion, and loosed him, and forgave him the debt.

"But the same servant went out, and found one of his fellowservants, which owed him an hundred pence [roughly $60]: and he laid hands on him, and took him by the throat, saying, Pay me that thou owest. And his fellowservant fell down at his feet, and besought him, saying, Have patience with me, and I will pay thee all. And he would not: but went and cast him into prison, till he should pay the debt.

"So when his fellowservants saw what was done, they were very sorry, and came and told unto their lord all that was done. Then his lord, after that he had called him, said unto him, O thou wicked servant, I forgave thee all that debt, because thou desiredst me: Shouldest not thou also have had compassion on thy fellowservant, even as I had pity on thee? And his lord was wroth, and delivered him to the tormentors, till he should pay all that was due unto him.

"So likewise shall my heavenly Father do also unto you, if

ye from your hearts forgive not every one his brother their trespasses" (Matt. 18:23–35).

The truth taught, then, is that the Lord is willing to forgive
us of our sins only if we are willing to forgive others of theirs.
The point is repeated in the Beatitudes: "Blessed are the merciful, for they shall obtain mercy" (Matt. 5:7).

The Lord's Prayer describes very clearly how obtaining forgiveness works: "And forgive us our debts, as we forgive our
debtors." Then Christ's very next words following the prayer
clarify the point further: "For if ye forgive men their trespasses,
your Heavenly Father will also forgive you. But if ye forgive not
men their trespasses, neither will your Father forgive your trespasses" (Matt. 6:12, 14–15). Could it be stated more clearly than
that?

"With What Measure Ye Mete . . ."

We ourselves decide the standard by which we will one day
be judged. The scriptures, taken literally, are replete with statements of this truth. The Savior taught the concept in Matthew
7:1-2: "Judge not, that ye be not judged. For with what judgment ye judge, ye shall be judged; and with what measure ye
mete, it shall be measured to you again."

Luke recorded, "Be ye therefore merciful, as your Father
also is merciful. Judge not, and ye shall not be judged; condemn
not, and ye shall not be condemned: forgive, and ye shall be forgiven . . . For with the same measure ye mete withal it shall be

measured to you again" (Luke 6:36–38).

If we demand justice from others, then justice will be demanded from us. If we do not judge with compassion, then we will not be judged with compassion. But, if we are merciful and forgiving of others, then God will extend his mercy to us and forgive our sins. And *that* is justice! What could be more just than to get back exactly what we give out?

Charity Covers a Multitude of Sins

Another exciting concept I learned was that if I possess charity, the Lord will overlook my own human frailties and imperfections. Once again, we must take the scriptures literally: "And above all things have fervent charity among yourselves; for charity shall cover the multitude of sins" (I Pet. 4:8). When I read that verse, I immediately became interested! Fervent charity—I liked that. It made me want to run out onto the street and call out, "I love you *all*, and I forgive *everybody!*"

In speaking of the woman who washed his feet with her tears and dried them with her hair, the Savior declared, "Her sins, which are many, are forgiven; for she loved much: but to whom little is forgiven, the same loveth little" (Luke 7:47). God extends his merciful forgiveness to us as we extend charity to others.

Charity and forgiveness go together; a person cannot possess one without the other.

"Be Ye Therefore Perfect"

The last verse of Matthew chapter 5 records Christ's injunction to "be ye therefore perfect, even as your Father which is in heaven is perfect."

Since sincere followers of Christ often read this scripture with feelings of guilt, thinking of their weaknesses and human frailties and imperfections, it was a happy day for me when I came to understand more fully what Christ was referring to when he gave this admonition. He was not discussing rigid obedience to rules or living the letter of the law. Rather, He was speaking of loving our enemies and the unconditional love of our Father in heaven, who "sends rain upon the just and the unjust and permits the sun to rise on the evil and on the good" (Matt. 5:45). God loves *all* of His children perfectly—whether they are deserving or not, whether they are worthy or not. Christ enjoined *us* to do the same—to bestow our love and forgiveness on everyone, regardless of whether or not they may seem to deserve it.

"Be *ye* therefore perfect, even as your Father in heaven is perfect." Impossible, you say? Were it not possible to love unconditionally, He would not have commanded it. Were it not possible to forgive those who have made themselves our enemies, He would not have commanded it. Were it not possible to "turn the other cheek," He would not have commanded it.

By gaining this charity—by learning to love and forgive despite what might have been done to us—we can become like our Father in heaven. We can be perfect, as He is.

"And above all these things put on *charity*, which is the bond of *perfectness*" (Col. 3:14, emphasis added).

Reflecting on his assignment to lead a world-wide church, the late Harold B. Lee recalled, "I came to a night some years ago, when upon my bed, I realized that if I would be worthy of the high place to which I had been called, I must love and forgive every soul that walks this earth."

With all due respect, I must say that *all* of us have been called to a "high place," even the Kingdom of Heaven. And *all* of us, in order to qualify, must "love and forgive every soul that walks this earth."

The words of Herbert carry new meaning for me: "He that cannot forgive others breaks the bridge over which he must pass himself, for every man has need to be forgiven."

O man, forgive thy mortal foe,
Nor ever strike him blow for blow;
For all the souls on earth that live,
To be forgiven must forgive.
Forgive him seventy times and seven,
For all the blessed souls in heaven
Are both forgivers and forgiven.
                              —ALFRED LORD TENNYSON

CHAPTER SEVEN
Loving Our Enemies

Always forgive your enemies:
nothing annoys them so much.
—UNKNOWN

T MAY SEEM to be a normal reaction, to pro-
tect oneself from an enemy. Broadly defined,
an enemy is anyone with the capability of hurting or doing us
harm. Common sense would suggest that one should defend
himself—even avenge himself— against a foe. But Jesus taught
otherwise:

"Ye have heard that it hath been said, Thou shalt love thy
neighbor, and hate thine enemy. But I say unto you, love your
enemies, bless them that curse you, do good to them that hate
you, and pray for them which despitefully use you, and persecute
you" (Matt. 5:43–44).

On the surface, His teachings seem to defy logic, to fly in
the face of reality. Christ's method of dealing with an enemy
would appear to be moral suicide, the feeblest surrender to
aggression. On the contrary, it is superb spiritual strategy.

"Christ said that when someone injures you, instead of
seeking to return the same to him, you are to do the opposite.
You are to forgive him and set him free. He knew that only then

can you be freed yourself; only then can you possess your own soul. To return evil for evil, to answer violence with violence, and hate with hate, is to start a vicious circle to which there is no ending but the wearing out of your own life and your brother's, too" (Emmet Fox, *The Sermon on the Mount*).

Perhaps we are waiting for those whom we perceive to have wronged us to come to us and apologize, to beg our forgiveness, offering to make amends. It would be so easy then to embrace them and say that all is forgiven. But what of those who never have and never will ask forgiveness, who deny any wrongdoing, refusing to even acknowledge the pain they have caused? Must we forgive them?

Here is an opportunity for us to be followers of Christ in deed as well as word. In fact, it may be a test of our true discipleship. "For if ye love them which love you, what reward have ye" (Matt. 5:46)?

Power in Humility

It requires meekness and humility to love and forgive an enemy. At some level, we may associate meekness with weakness. Yet, if extending forgiveness is for weaklings, then why is it so difficult, even impossible, for so many to do?

A man who had experienced death and then returned to life shared one of the insights he had gained: "Being humble doesn't mean being weak; it means to be strong. If you are humble, you are stronger than the strongest warrior of the world. We must lose ourselves to find ourselves. It is this new revelation, humbling ourselves . . . [and] loving our enemies . . . that will connect us with infinity."

As Mother Teresa said, "If you are humble, nothing will bother you, neither praise nor slander, because you know what you are."

In the scriptures we learn of a people who suffered "great persecutions" and "waded through much affliction." "Nevertheless, they did fast and pray oft, and did wax *stronger and stronger in their humility* . . . because of their yielding their hearts unto God" (Hel. 3:34–35).

Returning good for evil, offering love, mercy, and forgiveness rather than resistance—these are things that issue from a position of strength. They are not only acts of charity, but also acts of power. What can be more powerful than God extending his mercy and forgiveness to us? Can we feel a portion of such power when we do the same for others? This is exactly what we are commanded to do, if we want the promised blessings. "But love ye your enemies . . . and *your reward shall be great, and ye shall be the children of the Highest*: for he is kind unto the unthankful and to the evil" (Luke 6:35).

Emmet Fox spoke of the power in love when he said: "There is no difficulty that enough love will not conquer; no disease that enough love will not heal; no door that enough love will not open; no gulf that enough love will not bridge; no wall that enough love will not throw down; no sin that enough love will not redeem. . . . It makes no difference how deeply seated may be the trouble; how hopeless the outlook; how muddled the tangle; how great the mistake. A sufficient realization of love will dissolve it all. If only you could love enough you would be the happiest and most powerful being in the world. . . ."

Only love is powerful enough to destroy an enemy, for, as someone said, "The only safe and sure way to destroy an enemy is to make him your friend."

Returning Good for Evil

If you do not forgive, you become like your enemy. The only response to hatred is love; everything else will bring you down again.

"Live peaceably with all men . . . avenge not yourselves. . . . Therefore if thine enemy hunger, feed him; if he thirst, give him drink; for in so doing thou shalt heap coals of fire on his head. Be not overcome of evil, but overcome evil with good" (Romans 12:17–21).

Booker T. Washington was born into slavery and incredible poverty. He hungered for an education and, after the Civil War, obtained an education through great sacrifice. Later, he established Tuskegee Institute, an industrial school for blacks, became one of the most respected black men in his day, and was even awarded an honorary doctorate degree from Harvard.

An incident from his life interested me. One day Professor Washington was walking down the streets of Tuskegee. A woman failed to recognize him and said, "Come over here, boy, and chop this wood." So he chopped her wood and did a very good job.

As he walked away, the woman's servant recognized him.

"Why, that's Professor Washington," he said. "What was *he* doing here?"

The woman was mortified at her mistake. She finally mustered courage to visit him in his office, where she apologized for what she had done. "Why Madam," he replied, "I love to do favors for my friends."

Booker T. Washington understood the principle of overcoming evil with love. By so doing he "heaped coals of fire" on the head of his "enemy," allowing her own conscience to convict her. Nothing he could have said would have spoken louder than his love.

Truly, Booker T. Washington lived as he spoke: "I will not permit any man to narrow and degrade my soul by making me hate him."

O. C. Tanner shared his enlightened perspective: "Man is inclined to say that no one can love his enemy. This is because he *is* an enemy. An enemy cannot love his enemy. [But] a friend can love his enemy. A disciple of Jesus may *have* enemies; [but] he cannot *be* an enemy. We can love those who are wronging us. We cannot love those whom we are wronging."

My life was changed by C. Terry Warner's straightforward teachings. He maintains that when we resent someone, it is not because of the way he is treating us; it is because of the way we are treating *him*. "This lack of honesty with ourselves permits us to justify our own refusal to love. Elements of self-betrayal include blaming others, feeling hurt because of them, feeling threatened and defensive. Self-betrayers *need* others to be making trouble for them. They clutch at and cling to every evidence of wrongdoing on the part of the person they are blaming. It's their proof that [they are innocent]. They need trouble in order to feel justified in the way they are treating them" (*Bonds of Anguish, Bonds of Love*, excerpts).

"They Know Not What They Do"

Wayne Dyer shared his valuable insights: "Perhaps the picture of Christ forgiving those who are in the process of torturing and killing him is His most powerful utterance. 'Father, forgive them, for they know not what they do.' This is the very essence of Christianity, and yet very few are able to live up to these words.

"People who are inflicting harm on others really and truly do not know what they are doing to others. They are always acting out of their own feelings of anger and hatred. What they direct at others says nothing about the others. However, it says something very powerful about them. This is what you must learn about forgiveness. Those people who have behaved toward you in any way which you find hurtful really and truly do not know what they have done to you. . . . They are sending out their disharmony toward you because that is what they have to give away. Hating them for their behavior is akin to hating moss for growing on a tree and destroying the appearance of the tree. The moss only knows how to be moss, and regardless of your opinion about how it should not be behaving in such mosslike ways, it will still continue doing all that it knows how to do.

"Those who send out hatred are only acting out from where they are and how they have been thinking up until this moment. The enlightened person is sure enough of his own divineness that he does not judge himself in any negative manner because of the actions of others.

"Those who have hurt us truly know not what they do. For it is as true of anything I know about human beings that we cannot give away what we do not have, and we only give away what we do have. [That is why it has been said that "forgiveness is the fragrance a rose gives off when it is trampled upon."] If we give away hatred or harm in any way, it is because that is what we have. It is impossible for someone who has only love within to give away hatred. This is why your ability to forgive will come automatically when you truly become [Christlike, when you gain the pure love of Christ]" (*You'll See It When You Believe It,* excerpts).

With more compassion, we can see our enemies in a different light. Even the most depraved person started out as an innocent baby, a vulnerable little child, perhaps a wounded youth. You may not be able to change your oppressor with your love, but you can keep hatred from destroying your heart, mind, and life, as it has destroyed his.

Martin Luther King, Jr., once wrote about Jesus' command to forgive and love our enemies. "Forgiveness does not mean ignoring what has been done or putting a false label on an evil act. It means, rather, that the evil act no longer remains as a barrier to the relationship. . . . We must recognize that the evil deed

of the enemy neighbor, the thing that hurts, never quite express-
es all that he is. An element of goodness may be found even in
our worst enemy.

"The meaning of love is not to be confused with some sentimental outpouring. Love is something much deeper than emotional bosh. . . . Now we can see what Jesus meant when he said,
'Love your enemies.' We should be happy that he did not say,
'Like your enemies.' It is almost impossible to like some people.
'Like' is a sentimental and affectionate word. How can we be
affectionate toward a person whose avowed aim is to crush our
very being and place innumerable stumbling blocks in our path?
How can we like a person who is threatening our children or
bombing our homes? That is impossible. But Jesus recognized
that love is greater than like. When Jesus bids us to love our enemies, he is speaking of understanding and creative, redemptive
goodwill for all men. Only by following this way and responding
with this type of love are we able to be children of our Father
who is in heaven."

CHAPTER EIGHT

Forgiving Major Betrayals

The more we have been hurt,
the more we deserve to forgive.
—WENDY L. ULRICH

I T IS THE nature of mortality that we encounter opposition, that we experience pain and disappointment. We hurt others and are hurt by others, sometimes intentionally, sometimes not. In the give and take of everyday existence, people will occasionally injure our feelings, take unfair advantage, or be thoughtless or insensitive or ungrateful.

We can usually take the minor irritations in stride. But the serious hurts—betrayal or rejection by someone we trusted or someone close to us—may provide a difficulty of much greater magnitude. Indeed, it may be the greatest challenge of our lives.

Violent crimes, those actions that have robbed us of our innocence and childhood, serious abuses and major betrayals— surely these things would justify our being consumed by anger at the evil and the injustice of it all. To seek revenge might seem right, if not righteous.

A religious leader, Spencer J. Condie, spoke powerfully in regard to forgiving major betrayals. "Is an injured wife required to forgive her unfaithful husband? Yes! Are parents required to forgive their prodigal child who has besmirched their good family name? Yes! Are children required to forgive abusive parents? Yes! Must I really forgive a business associate who bilks me out of my pension? Yes!

"But where do we acquire the spiritual and emotional strength to forgive those who have offended us and sinned against us? The scriptures provide the prescription: 'Pray unto the Father with all the energy of heart, that ye may be filled with this love; . . . that when [Christ] shall appear we shall be like him; . . . that we may be purified even as he is pure' (Moro. 7:48).

"The goal of the great plan of happiness is to become like Christ so that we may someday dwell in his presence and in the presence of our Heavenly Father. An unforgiving and vengeful heart is unholy, as is the heart of an adulterer or someone addicted to pornography. Any inability we might have to forgive others becomes a barrier between us and the Savior. If we are to become like him, we must freely forgive others as he has forgiven us" ("The Fall and Infinite Atonement," *Ensign*, Jan. 1996, 27).

Healing by Forgiving

We would expect forgiveness for and healing from such evil imposed upon us to be difficult, if not impossible. At best, we might anticipate years of struggle as the natural process of grieving a loss is experienced. I used to believe that such suffering was not only understandable, but inevitable. Now I'm not so sure.

I have known and associated with many survivors of abuse—good people whose wounds go so deep and whose pain is so longstanding that it seems they will be affected their entire lives, that full recovery might be unattainable.

But with a proper understanding of forgiveness — knowing of its benefits and learning how to forgive, gaining a conviction of its freeing and healing power — I now believe that recovery is not only possible, it can be greatly expedited. Unencumbered and unfettered by the obsession with the evil that has been done to us, we find ourselves free to enjoy life and its abundant blessings. I believe that the miracle of forgiveness can take place, allowing us to experience a joy that we could not have imagined possible during those dark days of our initial anguish and agony. Healing can happen without wasting our lives in pain and suffering from the consequences of another's sinful choices and actions.

Forgiving does not minimize the evil. When we forgive depravity we do not excuse it, we do not tolerate it, we do not smother it. We look the evil full in the face, call it what it is, let its horror shock and stun and enrage us, and only then do we forgive it and move on with our lives. There is no real forgiving unless there is first acknowledgment.

Chieko Okazaki said, "Forgiveness is not the same thing as pretending that there's nothing to forgive. Great wrongs inspire deep indignation. It does no good to pretend that we are not angry when injustice, cruelty, or sheer stupidity destroys peace and happiness in our families and communities. We should not pretend that something doesn't matter or didn't hurt us when it *does* matter and it *did* hurt. But we also need to remember that forgiveness is one of the blessings that lies within God's gifts."

Wendy L. Ulrich spoke wisely when she said, "We *deserve* to forgive. In the eternities and in the present, inability to forgive interferes with our progress and our peace. The more we have been hurt, the more we deserve to forgive. Forgiveness is an opportunity to regain the internal peace of which evil has robbed us. . . . Forgiveness basically is a means of restoration to wholeness that the Spirit affords those victimized by others' actions" ("When Forgiveness Flounders: For Victims of Serious Sin," *Spiritual Recovery*).

In literature written for victims of abuse, it is said, "The best revenge is to live well." Surely, freeing oneself through forgiving qualifies as a very important way in which one can live well.

Forgiveness is a choice to cancel a debt; it is a pure act without anger or revenge, blame or guilt. Simply stated, one no longer allows the memory to hurt him further.

If we say that giants of evil are beyond forgiving, we give them a power they should never have. Those who seem too evil to be forgiven get a stranglehold on their victims, sentencing them to a lifetime of unhealed pain. If they are perceived as unforgivable monsters, they are given power to keep their evil alive in the hearts of those who suffered most. We give them power to condemn their victims to live forever with the hurting memory of their painful pasts. We give them the last word.

Instead, visualize yourself in the presence of the person who has violated you. Imagine yourself saying to him, "I forgive you for what you did." Then picture him saying to you, "Thank you. I set you free now."

Abuse

On the surface, it may seem unfair to be required to forgive someone who has so deeply violated us, oftentimes denying any wrongdoing. We want justice, and we want it NOW! Recently, the thought occurred to me that our insistence on justice in our own preferred time frame is simply a demonstration of a lack of faith in God. Can we not trust Him to be perfect in His justice as well as His mercy? Can we not trust Him to one day, in His own time, make everything right? Sometimes we must exercise patience, which is akin to faith. We can, with confidence, turn it over to God.

A religious leader, Vaughn J. Featherstone, spoke of incest, of justice and of trusting God. He said: "Those who have perpetrated great frauds and great deceit and abuse on others, may get out of this life without ever having confessed. The offending one can lie to ecclesiastical leaders—but they can't lie to the Spirit. Justice *will* take place.

". . . If you have been violated, if you have been abused as a child or as an adult, would you remember that we must forgive the offending one. We turn it over to God. It will not be left undone. We can have that absolute assurance. We must take it off our hearts.

"Some modern psychiatrists might say, 'Well, you don't get healed that way,' but you do. You do get healed by turning justice over to God and you forgiving. The Lord can lift all burdens from us. Once we turn it over to Him and simply say, 'It is between that person and God; I forgive,' then the burden will be lifted quietly and easily through the Savior's Atonement. That would only be just" (BYU Devotional Address, Sept. 1995).

One woman who had been sexually abused by her father wrote of her struggle to forgive him. "There were times when I interrogated myself mercilessly, asking how I could stand before God when my heart was filled with hatred. It seemed so basic. . . . This was Christianity at its core—'love one another.' This was a humbling experience for me. . . . But when I [finally] gave up and left it in God's hands, I felt free; it was no longer mine. . . .

"It seems so simple, almost too simple. But there are some things which are beyond us. At some point we have to let go and leave the unanswerable questions and conflicts to God. We leave these things in the hands of a God who understands forgiveness, but even more importantly a God who understands justice" (Sandra M. Flaherty, *Spirituality for Survivors of Childhood Sexual Abuse*, 138–139).

Another young woman, filled with malice toward her father because of childhood sexual abuse, was seemingly bent on self-destruction in her own life until she reached a point that she was able to forgive her father. She said, "I had never experienced happiness before, but now that I have, I will never go back."

She explained further. "I have really come to terms with what my dad did to me. I think part of it was that I knew that when he died he would have to feel the pain he had caused me and see the magnitude of his betrayal to me. And I wouldn't wish that on anyone, it is so deep. I know that he loved me in his own way, and it will kill him to really see what he did.

"I don't hate my father—I only feel sorrow for him, for the pain in his life that made him do those things to me. I forgive him. I am so happy." She freed herself by forgiving.

Marital Betrayals

"If I had my way," a wise old lawyer said, "I'd change the marriage promise to read, 'love, honor, and forgive.' It would be a healthy reminder of the power that could save many marriages."

In a magazine article the question was asked, "Should you forgive a major marital betrayal?" A marriage and family therapist responded, "If you're the one to forgive, it frees up the energy you have been devoting to anger. For the forgiven, it is powerful because it offers him a whole new motivation to change. He's facing the pain he caused you, and you're giving him another chance. If you don't forgive, there's a wall between the couple. The result is that one partner ends up perpetually bitter and angry and the other just gives up; the debt is too big to pay off."

Some who have been hurt by the transgression of a spouse express resentment and hatred, a spirit of revenge, saying that nothing that person could ever do would right the wrong he or she committed. A person with this attitude can hardly be termed a follower of Jesus Christ. Having the pure love of Christ—or charity—permits us to forgive those who do wrong.

One woman shared her experience and ensuing struggle after her husband's confession of infidelity. "My first reactions were completely in the Spirit. I could feel the love of Christ and Heavenly Father for my partner. In Their power and gift I could feel tender forgiveness and unconditional love carry me through that hour.

"Since then the moments have not all been as peaceful, I must admit. I find myself being tempted to get angry and be full of self-pity. I'm used to using my negative situations for my gain by sharing them with others so they will feel sorry for me and say things to me to justify my anger.

"I am finding, though, that it is a much calmer place to feel the comfort and what could be called justification of God. . . . Where I once would have announced to the world how wronged and victimized I've been, and let their cries for justice fan the fires and relieve me of all responsibility, I am now calling upon the name of my Savior. As I do, He takes my burdens and quietly helps me to keep the home fires burning. I am given the ability to nurture my children, accept my husband, and to feel an even greater hope in the Atonement of Christ than ever before. I know He has the ability to fix all that has been put out of place because of our sins.

". . . Other people's opinions and Satan's lies appeal to my pride and self-righteousness. He plants little thoughts like, 'I deserve better than this,' tempting me to ignore the fact that I have also sinned in serious ways and need to forgive as I would be forgiven. . . .

"Today, as I hold on to the Lord through this fiery pain in my heart I know that Christ is in my life in a way I have never known before, as I turn to Him in my need. He is my teacher, my Redeemer, my Savior, my Friend, my Beloved One. . . . I feel Him with me. I have finally come to know Jesus, and not just know *about* Him. I rejoice.

"His words speak to me in my heart and mind and urge me to accept the Atonement for my husband's sake and for my own sake. He urges me to believe that He loves my husband enough to redeem him from his sins, to forgive him just as wholeheartedly as He has forgiven me. I will believe in the hope of Christ" (*Heart t' Heart*).

When we follow Christ, we are able to help the weak to rise and then assist in sustaining them. In a personal account of his adultery and ultimate repentance, Steven Cramer tells in a poignant way the effects of charity and forgiveness through the eyes of the transgressor.

"I discovered God's love for his children through my family's forgiveness. From the moment of my confession, my selfless wife was able to look beyond her own pain to the needs of saving the family. I never felt a moment's revenge from her.

"Through the years of struggle, my family's attitude was that we were all in this together. Though I never deserved their love or forgiveness, their actions always affirmed: 'We still love you. We don't understand what you are going through, but it must be awful for you, and we want to help. We still need you, and we want you back as part of us. No matter how long this takes, you can count on us to see it through with you'" (*The Worth of a Soul*).

However, forgiving may not necessarily restore the trust that is vital to sustain a loving relationship. Forgiveness can mean hello or it can mean goodbye. Ongoing betrayals or continued abuse may dictate the appropriateness of ending a marriage. Yet we cannot emotionally detach ourselves from destructive relationships until we forgive those who have hurt us. Forgiveness is necessary in order to release ourselves to invest in new and, hopefully, healthier relationships. Otherwise, bitterness, resentments, and vengeful feelings are taken with us into new relationships where we are once again given the opportunity to deal with them. One day we *must* deal with them; we have no choice.

Violent Crimes

Richard Gayton recounted his journey to forgiveness after his wife was violently murdered in a robbery. "And just like that, after two years of waiting, [the trial] is over. . . . I should hate them for my wife's sake but . . . I have learned too much about the energy that rage takes from me. . . . I ask my inner guide what to do with the murderers.

They are your brothers.
They come from me as you have come from me.
What they do or what you do cannot change that.
They have joined you on a journey of forgiveness.
They to forgive themselves for what they have done.
You to no longer see what they have done.
You to see them for who they are, children of God,

So that you might see yourself for who you are.
Look beyond the rage and murder.
Look into the eyes of their souls and see yourself there
Waiting to be healed.
For your release is to release them.
There is no other way to peace.
Give this gift to yourself.

Unfortunately, he resisted his inner message, and his struggle continued: "I listen to my words, but I am not ready to let go. How could I? It would be disloyal to my wife's memory and let them off the hook somehow. There must be another way" ("Choosing Peace After Violent Trauma," *The Forgiving Place*, 21). Eventually, however, he learned that there is no other way, and he was able to let go and forgive.

The mother of one of the victims of the "hi-fi shop murders," at the time of the execution of one of the killers, said bitterly, "I hope his soul burns in hell forever."

Contrast that expression, understandable as it may be, with that of the mother of the 11-year-old Pocatello, Idaho, girl who was abducted on her paper route and murdered. After the mother thanked those who had helped in the search, she said, "I have learned a lot about love this week, and I also know there is a lot of hate. I have looked at the love and want to feel the love, and not the hate. We can forgive."

After the murder trial of O. J. Simpson, I observed the different attitudes of the families of the victims, the Browns (Nicole

Simpson's family) and the Goldmans. As they entered the court-room to hear the verdict, Mr. Brown had his arm around O. J. Simpson's mother. When asked about it later, he said, "She is a good Christian woman. It is so difficult for her to go through this at her age." His concern was for the mother of the accused murderer of his daughter.

After the verdict was delivered, Mr. Goldman, on the other hand, expressed his anger and bitterness that justice had not been served. The agitation felt by him is not hurting O. J. Simpson; it is hurting Mr. Goldman, preventing his own healing from the devastating event that cost him his son.

Another person learned about healing through forgiveness. A scientist spent four years as a slave laborer in Germany. His parents were killed by Nazi street bullies; his younger sister and older brother were sent to the gas chambers. This is a man who has every reason to hate. Yet he is filled with a love of life that he conveys to everyone who knows him. He explained: "In the beginning I was filled with hatred. Then I realized that in hating I had become my own tormentor. Unless you forgive, you cannot love. And without love, life has no meaning."

See the Offender for What He Is

Rather than viewing the person who has hurt us so deeply as a powerful monster, we can see him for what he is. We realize that he is a miserable, weak person trying desperately to feel stronger by overpowering and controlling others. Through different eyes, we can see his pain. We see his pathetic condition and feel sorrow and compassion for him. And even as we pity him, we know the power of Christ's Atonement can heal his wounds and make him whole. We can love him as the Savior would, when we see him as the Savior does.

To hate the sin yet love the sinner—this is more than a trite, overworked phrase. Not only is it the way of the Master, it is the way to our own spiritual peace and healing.

CHAPTER NINE

Forgiving Our Parents

*As we heal our past, we bridge
the gap between heaven and earth,
inviting God to come back to us.*
—UNKNOWN

IT IS NOT uncommon for grown children, raised by imperfect parents, to cling to resentments related to past events. We somehow expect parents to have anticipated and met our every need, and if they did not or could not, our judgment of them may be severe, our negative perceptions darkening our lives even in the present. But, as with any hurtful incident, what happened to us in the past is inconsequential compared to how we allow it to affect us now, in the present.

Love Holds No Grievances

Lynda Bates wrote: "All of our past relationships affect our present ones. If we think we can hold resentments toward one of our parents and fully love our children, we are fooling ourselves. The communication and true friendship we seek with our children are severely limited by our unwillingness to forgive our parents, or by our denial that we need to do so.

"We do not realize that our ability to love ourselves and others, and our ability to feel God's love, are all connected. If one of these relationships suffers, they all suffer. Likewise, we cannot heal one of these relationships without experiencing increasing intimacy in the others. . . . Jesus demonstrated with His life that we cannot hate some and love others and still understand love's meaning. Love holds no grievances. Unconditional love for those in our past and true intimacy in our present relationships cannot be experienced separately. They are a package deal.

"The intimacy within every relationship we have depends on our willingness to love and forgive as Jesus did—unconditionally and without exception."

The antithesis of this love and forgiveness was illustrated in the irony of a cartoon I saw. A woman standing beside a look-alike portrait of her mother was saying, "I hate my mother! She was so hateful! I'll never be like her!"

Terrence Olsen of the Department of Family Sciences at Brigham Young University, stated: "One of the most important things about memories is that we have to be living compassionately in the present to see, or even admit benefits from the past. If we are offended . . . we see things in the past as a source of pain that helps justify our current hardhearted attitude."

One woman's experience illustrates this point: "My grown son came one day to look through some family pictures I had copied for him. He chose to take all of them except the picture of my parents, his Grandpa and Grandma. He explained why, recalling his memory of a particular event years before: 'When I was about eight years old, Grandpa and Grandma were at our house. I had gone swimming or somewhere—with permission, of course. And I'm sure I came home on time—probably early, in fact. Grandma lit into me and told me I was wicked and going to hell—and ever since then, I haven't had much use for Grandma.'

The woman continued. "Just a couple of days later, I happened to stumble across my journal account of that event. My son's recollection and my journal account were so different. I had written: 'Mom said that while we were gone, she and Gordon [who was eleven years old] had had a run-in and he'd looked at her with a face filled with hatred and said, "You're just as mean as my mom!" And so she had told him everything she felt and thought about how he treated their daughter and how it hurt, as well as how his behavior (or misbehavior) was affecting the family. She cried. Then Dad [Grandpa], without having heard what Mom had said, repeated the same things.'"

Seeing the diversity in the two accounts, one might wonder if both Gordon and his grandmother might have used the event to feel justified in their mutual lack of love. Each may see the other as the source of the trouble in their relationship. "When we see the other person as the source of the problem, then that *is* the problem!"

Terrence Olsen's statement bears repeating: "One of the most important things about memories is that we have to be living compassionately in the present to see, or even admit benefits from the past. If we are offended . . . we see things in the past as a source of pain that helps justify our current hard-hearted attitude."

I like Ethel's words to her daughter, Chelsea, in *On Golden*

Pond: "Here we go again. You had a miserable childhood. . . . What else is new? Don't you think everyone looks back on their childhood with some bitterness or regret about something? You have this unpleasant chip on your shoulder which is very unattractive. . . . Life marches by; I suggest you get on with it."

Rewriting History

Forgiveness is the key that unlocks childhood pain, allowing us to heal. If we have harbored resentments toward a parent, it is not too late to "rewrite history"—to go back in our memories and review the hurtful event with a different, more compassionate perspective.

As a little boy, Gene Hackman watched his father drive out of his life. He was playing in the street and his father drove past him, offering only a slight wave of his hand. Instinctively, Gene somehow knew that that would be the last time he would see his father.

It wasn't until he was a grown man, established in his career as an actor, that Gene Hackman was finally able to meet with his father to confront him with his abandonment and the painful issues it had created in his life. But his father refused to talk about the past; he would speak only of the present and the future.

It was then that Gene realized that he and his father could relate now as two grown men. He saw that he should now be able to perceive the circumstances of his father's leaving with the perspective and the understanding of an adult rather than through the eyes of a pain-filled child. He could forgive his father.

The Apostle Paul said it: "This one thing I do, forgetting those things which are behind, and reaching forth unto those things which are before" (Philip. 3:13).

A personal experience illustrates the procedure of rewriting history with increased compassion. On one occasion, I was invited to recall an unresolved event from my past. My mind went back to 1969, the year I graduated from high school. It was also the year that I had won the title, "Miss FBLA" for Idaho, which qualified me to compete at the national FBLA (Future Business Leaders of America) convention in Dallas, Texas.

Although my self-confidence was actually extremely low, I was a good actress, and the results of my test scores, coupled with the interviews with the judges, brought me the honor of winning second place in the nation, first-runner-up to "Miss Future Business Leader of America." It was a thrill beyond my wildest hopes to have done so well competing against other girls who seemed so beautiful and so well qualified.

Later, when the awards banquet was over, I went to my hotel room and called home to share the exciting news, anticipating that my mother would be similarly elated. Her response surprised and hurt me as she said in a disappointed voice, "Oh, I have been waiting all day expecting to hear that you had won."

I was crushed. I thought, "Even winning second place in the nation is not good enough to satisfy my mother."

Now, many years later, I returned to that painful memory and "rewrote history" with more compassion. I had felt resentful that my mother apparently thought of me as an extension of herself, perhaps hoping for me to win honors and awards as a reflection on her.

Now I gave up those feelings that I had harbored, perceiving her with more charity: Why shouldn't she want those things for me? She had married at the age of 18, poor health having prevented her from finishing high school. She had gone through a great deal of pain and sacrifice, even against medical advice, to give birth to eight children. Her poor health and challenging finances and living conditions (we all lived in a one-bedroom house) had made life a struggle for her. After five boys, I had been her first daughter. Would it not be natural for her to want for her daughter opportunities for experiences that she had never had?

Now I also remembered her excitement for me as I had boarded the plane in Boise, flying to Dallas on my first plane ride. I thought, too, of the beautifully tailored suits she had painstakingly sewn for me so I would be dressed appropriately for the contest.

And even her disappointing response to my excited phone call I could now perceive in a different way. Rather than thinking that I was unable to satisfy my mother, I thought of it as a compliment that she apparently felt I was qualified enough to merit winning first place.

"Many of us allow ourselves to be hurt, to feel injured, to feel misunderstood. In our narrow vision of life, how many times do we make our own unhappiness and sorrow? . . . In these moments we have forgotten the message and example of the Savior. We have much need for forgiveness and need to forgive.

Only then can we heal or be healed." (Marjorie Luke)

With More Understanding

The account of Eileen Starr may be helpful. Her mother dutifully cooked meals for her and her sister and bought their clothes, but the children "felt deprived—emotionally deprived—by our mother. As adults, we have endlessly discussed the lack of warmth, approval . . . moral training, and hospitality . . . in our home. Why was Mother . . . uncaring, critical, and self-centered?"

Eileen was mothered by other women, but the hurt lingered even after her mother's death. Then one day, after weeping from her sorrow, she had an experience in which "a healing balm . . . washed away all of my bitterness and longing. I saw Mother, stalwart and whole. I was filled with the awareness that my mother had been handicapped in mortal life. She had had an emotional handicap, the source of which remains a secret to me. But she is handicapped no longer. And neither am I.

"Now," she says, "how thankful I am for the Savior and for His love, which extends to me and to my now-whole mother, who is learning the lessons she could not learn in mortal life. I am eager to meet her and to share the love with her we both were deprived of on earth" ("Forgiving My Mother," *Ensign*, Aug. 1990, 49).

It has been suggested that our own healing may be facilitated by visualizing self, mother, and father as children. Even as you feel sympathy and pity for yourself as a little child experiencing harsh treatment, you may also feel a similar sorrow and compassion when you visualize your parents as innocent, vulnerable little children, experiencing insensitivity or cruelty at the hands of others. See the pain in their eyes. Imagine holding and comforting them on your lap, wiping away their tears. You may feel more understanding of the way they treated you, more lenient in your judgment, more forgiving, as you contemplate the wounds of your childhood — and theirs.

We can recognize that they did the best they could with the knowledge and experience that they had. It is a worthy goal to wish to improve over the parenting that we may have received. In our desire to improve our future and the lives of our children, let us also remember to model for them charity and compassion for others, especially those closest to us.

As someone said, "Having learned to forgive, we know that life is lived forward, fueled by the energy of past forgiveness."

CHAPTER TEN

Let It Go

*The starting point of all change
is a willing mind.*
—UNKNOWN

I AM WRITING THIS chapter at the end of an old year and the start of a new one. It is a time of new beginnings, of new resolutions. Usually these resolutions take the form of positive additions to our lives: reading the scriptures more consistently, praying more fervently, beginning to exercise (again)! But here I shall deal with the opposite; not only starting new things, but letting go of some old ones.

Neal A. Maxwell said, "The pathway of discipleship is the only pathway where littering is permissible, even encouraged." Today I write of leaving behind debris, dropping it, letting it go.

At the new year, we are reminded of the words written by Alfred Lord Tennyson:

*Ring out, wild bells, to the wild sky,
The flying cloud, the frosty light.
The year is dying in the night;
Ring out, wild bells, and let him die.*

Ring out the old; ring in the new.
Ring, happy bells, across the snow.

The year is going; let him go.
Ring out the false; ring in the true.

Ring in the valiant men and free,
The larger heart, the kindlier hand.
Ring out the darkness of the land;
Ring in the Christ that is to be.

Quality of Life

A number of years ago, I wrote some articles about growing older. I interviewed several elderly people and found most of them to have happy, positive attitudes. One woman, however, seemed to revel in recounting to me every offense that had come to her in life. She recalled all the pain that had been the result of others' mistreatment of her. Her feelings toward her grown children were bitter and she was filled with resentment, her judgment of them blaming and accusative. She expressed a hope that one day her life could be made into a movie; it had been so exceptionally fraught with undeserved heartache. It appeared that the accumulation of the hurts was a great and heavy burden for her. Considering herself to be a victim, she seemed miserable indeed.

A time for healing—why not now? How much happier

would we find ourselves, free of the burden of old wounds, old grudges, old judgments and negative feelings. Why drag dead wood, scars, and thorns with us into our future—the future that we create for ourselves? To be wronged is irrelevant unless we continue to remember it.

Resentments can be very deceiving. We may think we have dealt with them, when instead of letting go, we have carefully packed them away or buried them. Yet, feelings buried alive never die. They lie in our subconscious, continuing to cause anger, hostility, and discontent.

Forgiveness is not a form of denial, a means of avoiding. It allows us to release that which was once held. Forgiveness does not undo what has been done; it enables us to accept what has happened and go on from there.

As with all forms of surgery, spiritual surgery may be painful. But it is a healing kind of pain that can be worked through. Furthermore, once the letting go is complete, a healthier person emerges; one with a straight back, a lighter heart, and a freer, more peaceful spirit, one who knows he is capable of forgiving.

From Turmoil to Peace

Recently, a woman telephoned me after reading one of my first booklets on forgiveness. She was distraught as she confessed, "I'm still having trouble letting go!"

We must have been on the telephone for over an hour. She began by explaining the nature of the major transgressions that had been committed against her by her former husband. Surely she felt justified in her bitter feelings; her complaints were valid, her suffering real. "But I hate how I am feeling!" she said. She told, too, of how her relationship with her children was suffering because of her rancor—of how they felt a need to defend their father to her. She felt no peace. I sympathized as I remembered my own earlier struggle and how I had clung to my pain and had been obsessed by it, feeling a need to share it with others. How grateful I felt to be past that!

I could tell this was a good woman. Perhaps Satan could not tempt her to be immoral or to rob a bank or commit other major transgressions. So if he couldn't bring her down one way, he could try another—and this hardness of heart and failure to forgive was potentially more devastating to her eternal future than any other sin might be. "For that same spirit which doth possess your bodies at the time that ye go out of this life, that same spirit will have power to possess your body in that eternal world" (Alma 34:34). There will be no bitter, vengeful spirits in heaven.

Surely, she wished to let it go. The inner conflict and turmoil and strife she was experiencing were debilitating her.

"For where envying and strife is, there is confusion and every evil work. But the wisdom that is from above is first pure, then peaceable, gentle, and easy to be entreated, full of mercy and good fruits, without partiality, and without hypocrisy. And the fruit of righteousness is sown in peace of them that make peace" (James 3:16–18).

As a person struggles with forgiveness, peace is the one commodity most lacking, it seems. Thus, the scripture's promise of peace is most encouraging. "As the elect of God, put on mercy, kindness, humbleness of mind, meekness, longsuffering, . . . forgiving one another, if any man have a quarrel against any: even as Christ forgave you, so also do ye. And above all these things put on charity, which is the bond of perfectness. And let the peace of God rule in your hearts" (Col. 3:12–15).

Hanging On or Letting Go

Two stories illustrate the consequences of choosing to hang on or to let go. The first is about a man who was walking along the street one day and bent over to pick up a piece of string. Someone saw him and accused him of taking money or a wallet that did not belong to him. He was arrested and taken to jail. The error was soon discovered and he was released. Truly, he had been unfairly treated. The embittered man told everyone he met about the episode. It continued to fester inside him for the rest of his life. At his death, the last words he uttered were, "a piece of string."

In contrast to that story was one shared in an address by Boyd K. Packer. He prefaced his telling of the story by saying, "My message is an appeal to those who are not at peace, those whose lives are touched with bitterness, with hostility, or with resentment. It is a plea to those who anxiously struggle. . . . We see so much unnecessary suffering, so many who cripple themselves spiritually carrying burdens which could be put down. Many suffer from real misfortune and injustice. Sadly, some only imagine that they do. In either case, self-inflicted penalties soon become cruel and unusual punishment. . . .

"Consider this lesson taught to me many years ago by an older man — as saintly a man as I have ever known. He was steady and serene, with a deep spiritual strength that many drew upon. . . . On one occasion he gave me a lesson for my life from an experience in his own. . . .

"He grew up in a little community with a desire to make something of himself. He struggled to get an education. He married his sweetheart. They were deeply in love, and she was expecting their first child.

"The night the baby was to be born, there were complications. The only doctor was somewhere in the countryside tending to the sick. After many hours of labor, the condition of the mother-to-be became desperate. Finally the doctor was located. In the emergency, he acted quickly and soon had things in order. The baby was born and the crisis, it appeared, was over. Some days later, the young mother died from the very infection that the doctor had been treating at another home that night.

"John's world was shattered. . . . As the weeks wore on, his grief festered. 'That doctor should not be allowed to practice,' he would say. 'He brought that infection to my wife. If he had been careful, she would be alive today.'

"He thought of little else, and in his bitterness, he became threatening. Today, no doubt, he would have been pressed by many others to file a malpractice suit. . . . But that was another day, and one night a knock came at his door. A little girl said simply, 'Daddy wants you to come over. He wants to talk to you.' A grieving, heartbroken young man went to see his spiritual leader. This spiritual shepherd had been watching his flock and had something to say to him.

"The counsel from that wise servant was simply, 'John, leave it alone. Nothing you do about it will bring her back. Anything you do will make it worse. John, leave it alone.'

"My friend told me then that this had been his trial—his Gethsemane. How could he leave it alone? Right was right! A terrible wrong had been committed and somebody must pay for it. It was a clear case. But he struggled in agony to get hold of himself. And finally, he determined that whatever else the issues were, he should be obedient. . . . He would leave it alone.

"Then he told me, 'I was an old man before I understood! It was not until I was an old man that I could finally see a poor country doctor—overworked, underpaid, run ragged from patient to patient, with little medicine, no hospital, few instruments, struggling to save lives, and succeeding for the most part.

"'He had come in a moment of crisis, when two lives hung in the balance, and had acted without delay. I was an old man,' he repeated, 'before I finally understood! I would have ruined my life,' he said, 'and the lives of others.' Many times he had thanked the Lord on his knees for a wise spiritual leader who counseled simply, 'John, leave it alone.'

"And that is the counsel I bring again to you," continued Packer. "If you have a festering grudge, if you are involved in an acrimonious dispute, 'Behold what the scripture says [and it says it fifty times and more]—man shall not smite, neither shall he judge; for judgment is mine, saith the Lord, and vengeance is mine also, and I will repay' (Morm. 8:20).

"Some frustrations we must endure without really solving the problem. Some things that ought to be put in order are not put in order because we cannot control them. Things we cannot solve, we must survive. If you resent someone for something he has done—or failed to do—forget it. . . .

"We call this forgiveness. Forgiveness is powerful spiritual medicine. To extend forgiveness, that soothing balm, to those who have offended you is to heal. And more difficult yet, when the need is there, forgive yourself. I repeat, 'Leave it alone.'

"Purge and cleanse and soothe your soul and your heart and your mind and that of others. A cloud will then be lifted, a beam cast from your eye. There will come that peace which surpasseth understanding" ("Balm of Gilead," *Ensign*, Nov. 1987, 16–18).

For Our Own Sake

Even God himself lets go and forgives for his own sake: ". . . thou hast wearied me with thine iniquities. I, even I, am he that blotteth out thy transgressions *for mine own sake*, and will not remember thy sins" (Isaiah 43:24–25, emphasis added).

Imagine how miserable the Lord would be if he held grudges and harbored bitter, hard feelings against everyone who offended him? Everyone who took his name in vain, everyone who flaunted his counsel and his commandments, everyone who rejected his love, refused his offerings, everyone who hurt him or his beloved children in any way? He would be most miserable. So, for his own sake, he lets it go.

If It Isn't Love, Let It Go

Louise Hay speaks and writes of healing and forgiveness: "There is something we can do to open the doorway to love so that love can flow most abundantly in our lives. We can forgive. When the doorway to love seems to be stuck, it is usually because there is something or someone we are unwilling to forgive. Yes, it may be true that we have had a very unpleasant experience in our past. That is unfortunate, but it is not unforgivable.

"Forgiveness is a gift to ourselves, for it sets us free. When we refuse to forgive, we sit in a prison of self-righteous resentments and stay stuck in the past. This hurts only ourselves. The other person may not even know we are in pain.

"If you really wanted to forgive . . . you know you could. What is it you want to hold onto? Would you rather be right, or would you rather be happy? Perhaps you have held [onto] this pain long enough. And now it is safe enough for you to let it go. What would you be willing to give in return for releasing this negative feeling? Could you give understanding for abandonment? Could you now give compassion for the old abuse and betrayal? Could you give acceptance for rejection? Could you just forgive and let go?

"Are you willing to change your old beliefs? How willing are you to give up old ideas for a new freedom that forgiveness can give you?

"Once again, just release all of this pain, drop all of this bitterness—let it go, release it, set it free. Say, 'I forgive you for not being the way I wanted you to be. I forgive you and I set you free.' Set yourself free of every vestige of the past. You are cleansed and you are free. . . .

"The weight has been taken away. What a relief! What a joy! Feel the space opening up in your heart. Feel the love beginning to flow. There is nothing to stop it now. You feel so peaceful, so relaxed, so alive, so willing to love, so very free. You have forgiven and you have been forgiven."

We often think of repentance as a long, drawn-out process. In truth, we can repent in a fraction of a second. Repentance simply means a change of direction, a change of heart—and that can happen in an instant. Of course we will want to spend the rest of our lives demonstrating our repentance, but the actual act, that change of heart, can occur instantly. Search your heart now for the injustices you still carry, then let them go.

And so, at this new year, this time of new beginnings, this is my wish for you:

To leave the old with a burst of song,
To recall the right and forgive the wrong,
To forget things that bind you fast,
To the vain regrets of the year that's past.
To have the strength to let go your hold
Of the not worthwhile of the days grown old,
To dare go forth with a purpose true,
To the unknown task of the year that's new.

To help your brother along the road,
To do his work, and lift his load,

To add your gift to the world's good cheer,
Is to have, and to give—a Happy New Year!

—AGNES FOTH

CHAPTER ELEVEN

Life Is Too Short to Be Little

*Life appears to me too short to be spent in
nursing animosity or registering wrong.*
—CHARLOTTE BRONTE

W E CHOOSE OUR own quality of life.
There are consequences for every act, every
thought. If we live one way, we'll get one result. Every person is
a product of the dominating thoughts he permits to occupy his
mind. We ought to be smart enough, aware enough, realistic
enough, and observant enough to realize this.

The past and the future exist only in our thoughts. *Now* is
the only time we really have. Without forgiveness, we are con-
stantly living in the past or fearing the future. We fail to live in
and enjoy the present.

Disraeli said it beautifully. "Life is too short to be little.
There are too many worthwhile causes to serve, too many great
books, lectures, musicals, trips, friends, loved ones to help—too
much to be little—grumbling over past painful experiences,
brooding over injuries, conjuring up ways to get even, smarting
over grievances until we cannot sleep. Life is too short."

André Maurois similarly observed, "Often we allow ourselves to be upset by small things we should despise and forget.

Perhaps some man we helped has proved ungrateful . . . some woman we believed to be a friend has spoken ill of us . . . some reward we thought we deserved has been denied us. We feel such disappointments so strongly that we can no longer work or sleep. But isn't that absurd? Here we are on this earth, with only a few more decades to live, and we lose many irreplaceable hours brooding over grievances that, in a year's time, will be forgotten by us and by everybody. No, let us devote our life to worthwhile actions and feelings, to great thoughts, real affections and enduring undertakings. For life is too short to be little."

Life is too brief
Between the budding and the falling leaf,
Between the seed time and the golden sheaf,
For hate and spite.
We have no time for malice and for greed;
Therefore, with love make beautiful the deed;
Fast speeds the night.

Life is too swift
Between the blossom and the white snow's drift,
Between the silence and the lark's uplift,
For bitter words.
In kindness and in gentleness our speech
Must carry messages of hope, and reach
The sweetest chords.

Life is too great
Between the infant's and the man's estate

Between the clashing of earth's strife and fate,
For petty things.
Lo! We shall yet who creep with cumbered feet
Walk glorious over heaven's golden street.
Or soar on wings!

—W. M. VORIES

I love the sobering thoughtfulness expressed by Joseph Addison more than 250 years ago. "When I look upon the tombs of the great, every emotion of envy dies in me; when I read the epitaphs of the beautiful, every inordinate desire goes out; when I meet with the grief of parents upon a [child's] tombstone, my heart melts with compassion, [but] when I see the tombs of the parents themselves, I consider the vanity of grieving for those whom we must quickly follow; when I see kings lying by those who deposed them, when I consider rival wits placed side by side, or the men that divided the world with their contests and disputes, I reflect with sorrow and astonishment on the little competitions, factions, and debates of mankind. When I read the several dates of the tombs, of some that died yesterday, and some six hundred years ago, I consider that great Day when we shall all of us be contemporaries, and make our appearance together."

Quality of Life

What quality of life do you want for yourself? "There is an old woman up there ahead of you, and you ought to know her.

She looks somewhat like you, talks like you, walks like you. She has your nose, your eyes, your chin. And whether she loves you or hates you, respects you or despises you, whether she is miserable or happy depends on you, for *you* made her. She is you, grown older." (Unknown)

Things happen that can either ruin our lives or give us opportunities for growth. When we choose to forgive, we are making the choice to move from hatred and despair to love and joy.

All of us wish to be happy, to lead lives of fulfillment. Someone said, "One of the secrets of a long and fruitful life is to forgive everybody everything every night before you go to bed." Fill each day and each hour with happy memories, happy thoughts, and things that will be of value in our eternal lives.

We cannot be happy as long as we live in a world of fear and hatred. Release from fear and hatred comes only through forgiveness. The unforgiving heart, contrasted with the forgiving heart, is confused, afraid, and full of fear. Forgiveness is the key to happiness. Forgiveness is the only road to peace.

Our Father in heaven and our elder brother, Jesus Christ, are one in purpose. They are unified in their desire to ultimately see us happy. While studying the beatitudes, I learned the original meaning of the word *blessed,* the word with which each beatitude begins. *Blessed,* translated, means *happy* in most modern versions. In Hebrew, blessed means more literally, *Oh, the happiness of.* The Greek word means, *O how divinely happy.* Indeed, the entire aim of the Beatitudes is to show the best and most joyous way of living. The fact that Christ begins each beatitude with this word indicates how eager he was for people to be happy.

His teachings were intended for those who suffer from the insults of life. He asked people to live above offenses. Christ set forth a way of life that acclaims the meek, forgiving man—one who returns good for evil, even in the face of mistreatment, injustice, and cruelty from others.

Why are the scriptures replete with admonitions for us to forgive? Because it is the way to peace and happiness and healing. Jesus knows that, and we must trust Him enough to follow His teachings, and then we will know it, too.

"After you let go of hurt and resentment through forgiveness, the void is filled by such things as serenity, gratitude, self-respect, and kindness. Forgiveness provides the spirit with room to grow. As it grows, the spirit becomes stronger. The bitterness is replaced by warmth. . . . Forgiveness does not take you back to the person you were before you were hurt. It takes you to a much higher plane" (Robert J. Furey, *The Joy of Kindness*, 91–92).

Forgiveness does not change the past, but it does enlarge our future. We can consciously choose the thoughts that we allow to fill our minds, our hearts, our lives. There are two things we should learn to forget: the good we have done to others, and the evil they have done to us. Unfortunately, many of us remember the things we should forget, and forget the things we should remember.

A Memory System

Forget each kindness that you do as soon as you have done it,
Forget the praise that falls to you the moment you have won it,
Forget the slander that you hear before you can repeat it,

Forget each slight, each spite, each sneer,
Wherever you may meet it.

Remember every kindness done to you whate'er its measure,
Remember praise by others won and pass it on with pleasure,
Remember every promise made and keep it to the letter,
Remember those who lent you aid, and be a grateful debtor.

Remember all the happiness that comes your way in living;
Forget each worry and distress; be hopeful and forgiving.
Remember good, remember truth,
Remember heaven's above you,
And you will find through youth and age,
True joys, and hearts to love you.

—UNKNOWN

Forgive and Forget

Don't let old grievances canker your soul and destroy love and life. If we wish to be happy, we must rid ourselves of resentment and pettiness and foolish pride; we must choose to love and to forgive.

Let us use a hypothetical situation to see how our own quality of life is affected by the things that we allow to upset us. Suppose you have driven into the crowded parking lot of a busy store. You are glad to see a parking space being vacated near the entrance and position your car to take the spot as soon as the other car is out of the way. But, before you can take action, another vehicle whips around the corner and into the spot you had planned to take.

Suppose you enter the store fuming at the wrong done to you, indignant at the injustice, angry at the utter selfishness and crass insensitivity of the individual who had robbed you of your intended parking space. Your stomach is churning. Your blood pressure rises. It is difficult for you to concentrate on the list of groceries you'd come for.

You enter each store aisle with dreaded anticipation, fearing a possible meeting with the person who had trespassed against you—expecting either an angry confrontation or the necessity for a hasty retreat and thus avoidance of crossing paths with him, depending on your personality type.

Furthermore, in your mind, the thoughtless action of that individual has been the cause of your feelings of irritability toward others—shoppers who are in your way, folks ahead of you in the checkout line, the slow checker.

Meanwhile, the person who offended you is blithely shopping, happily selecting his cereal and juice, totally oblivious to your miserable state. And you, stewing in your own juices, have allowed negative feelings to consume you! Whose quality of life suffers when we focus our thoughts and energies on the injustices done to us?

We can consciously choose a better way. We can achieve a positive focus in our lives, one that brings happiness.

If you were busy being kind,
  Before you knew it, you would find
You'd soon forget to think t'was true,
  That anyone was unkind to you!

If you were busy being glad,
  And cheering people who were sad,
Although your heart did ache a bit,
  You'd soon forget to notice it.

If you were busy being good
  And doing just the best you could,
You'd soon forget to blame the man
  For doing just the best he can.

If you were busy being right,
  You'd be yourself too busy quite,
To criticize your neighbor long,
  Because he's busy being wrong.
    —UNKNOWN

What could you want that forgiveness cannot give? Do you want peace? Forgiveness offers it. Do you want happiness, a feeling of safety and comfort and warmth that cannot be disturbed? Forgiveness bestows all this upon you, and more. When you awaken, it gives you joy to meet the day. It soothes you while you sleep and rests upon you, removing all dreams of fear, evil, and malice. And when you wake again, it offers you another day of harmony and serenity.

A friend wrote this spring of his exuberance for life. "I'm thrilled to see spring coming. Winter can be wonderful, fall is fun, and summer is super, but for me, spring is spectacular. It is the season of hope—proof that a long, dark, cold spell will eventually succumb to warmth, light, and life. Soon the days will be warmer, the sun will be out longer, the birds will sing in the morning, and everything will be green.

"The Savior tells us that he is 'the light and the life of the world.' This being so, then spring is the season of the Savior. How fitting that Easter, the celebration of physical and spiritual rebirth, comes as herald to proclaim the advent of spring. What a perfect time to renew friendships, to seek new friends, to forgive grievances, to seek forgiveness ourselves, to repair strained relationships, and to 'make old things new.'"

Francis Bernardone was born in Assisi in the late 1100's. He was a spoiled child, doted on by his wealthy parents. As he grew older, much of his time was wasted in pleasure seeking and lascivious living. He had always wanted to be a knight; however, he began to learn of a different life's mission.

He made dramatic changes in his life, becoming more sensitive to others, especially the plight of the poor. He denounced his previous life of ease, becoming a beggar, but he was completely free. He became a monk, preaching of God's love. One observer wrote: "This coarsely dressed monk with a cord around his waist who made his audience weep and sigh was someone they had seen four years ago when he was the king of youth, wasting his father's money in aristocratic style and living in disorder and sensuality."

Today we know him as Saint Francis of Assisi. He learned of the things that really matter. He knew of the qualities that bring true joy in this temporary, transitory state of being we call life. By his attitudes and actions he demonstrated his belief that "life is too short to be little." His words have become immortal. We, too, might do well to write them on our hearts.

Lord, make me an instrument of Thy peace;
Where there is hatred, let me sow love;
Where there is injury, pardon;
Where there is doubt, faith;
Where there is despair, hope;
Where there is darkness light;
Where there is sadness, joy;

O Divine Master, grant that I may not so much seek
To be consoled as to console,
To be understood as to understand,
To be loved as to love;

For it is in giving that we receive.
It is in pardoning that we are pardoned;
It is in dying that we are born to eternal life.

CHAPTER TWELVE

Our Best Teachers

*Everyone who came into your life
was a teacher. . . . There truly
are no accidents. . . .*

—WAYNE DYER

I F WE COULD see the entire picture, perhaps we
would look upon our past with gratitude rather
than resentment—gratitude for the important lessons all our
brothers and sisters have taught us.

Wayne Dyer assures us, "Everything that happened to you
is a lesson you can be grateful for. Everyone who came into your
life was a teacher, regardless of how much you choose to hate and
blame him or her. There truly are no accidents. . . . All of those
situations, including when you were a small child, contain
immensely valuable lessons for you to absorb and benefit from,
lessons which are blocked by feelings of hate and blame."

Memories Can Serve Us

Cato Jaramillo was only 12 when the Nazis put her in a
labor camp under the worst conditions imaginable. But even
before that, she experienced a home life bereft of love. Unwanted
and abused, she lived with an alcoholic father and a caustic, cold

mother. "I will never forget my childhood, as hard as I tried for many years. I tried to forget walking around in rags, with holes in my socks and scuffed up shoes. I tried to forget the house I never wanted to go home to. I tried to forget wanting love I could not have. Yet in an odd sort of way, that childhood prepared me for what was to come later in life. What a strange reason to be thankful to my parents—their callousness toughened me enough to survive the cruelty I would later know" (*Too Stubborn to Die*, 8).

Today Cato speaks to young people about the possible consequences of hatred and violence. She speaks of overcoming her own hatred: "I have carried with me memories of things unknown to most people, but I have not allowed those memories to poison my life. Horrible memories can be the best teachers we have. They can keep us from ever creating the same memories for another human being. I will never allow myself to forget mine.

"My memories are my salvation. They have tamed my soul and kept me from being able to hurt anyone weaker than I. They rise up within me and restrain my hands, soften my voice, and help me see with compassion. Your memories do not have to rule you—they can serve you. They can create in you a heart so kind that you cry out in defense of the helpless and harmless. Your memories of pain do not excuse you from becoming strong and loving human beings" (*Too Stubborn to Die*, x–xi).

A child's story further illustrates. The ugly duckling was persecuted and ridiculed by his brothers and sisters in the barnyard. He could have harbored bitter resentments for the cruel way in which he had been treated by his siblings. He could have blamed them for any unhappiness he might feel in the present, for any difficulties he might be experiencing now. Since he had grown into a beautiful swan and the tables were turned, he could have taken revenge and mocked them just as they had earlier mocked him.

Instead, he turned it into a growing experience, feeling gratitude for the lessons he had learned: "Now I know how it feels to be treated that way," he said, "and I will never, ever treat anyone else in that way!"

I have often observed that the people who demonstrate the greatest compassion and sensitivities are those who seem to have experienced the most grief. Even as I write, I sit here with two broken legs, the result of osteoporosis. Although one leg had been incredibly painful and swollen for a month, the fracture was not discovered until the second leg snapped and both legs were X-rayed.

In the following days I was visited repeatedly by my neighbor. She brought over her "boot" for me to borrow, for she had just recovered from a badly broken leg herself. She sent over a casserole for us and another time came to spend some time with me, bringing muffins.

In the course of our conversation, she revealed that she had received few visits or calls during the time she was bedridden with her broken leg. Additionally, two years earlier, after discovering in the same week that her husband had cancer and that her son had a large brain tumor, both requiring radical surgery, she recalled the initial surge of sympathy from others and then her feelings of abandonment when the expressions of concern ceased. She did not want me to experience the same feelings. Rather than allowing it to canker her soul, make her become bitter and turn inward, she was willing to learn from this "teacher," allowing her own pain to make her more sensitive to the feelings and needs of others.

Learning from Our Suffering

Do we really think we are here on earth just to watch other people hurt — to learn from *their* suffering and not our own? We came here to learn from our *own* experiences, painful as they may be. This learning process may appear to be unfair, as the innocents seem to suffer disproportionately. But if we are willing to let him, God can work all these things together for our own good.

The great tragedy of this life is not in suffering, but suffering in vain. It is only wasted if we learn nothing by it. Terrence Olsen stated, "Our richest storehouse of understanding is our own experience. We actually learn a great deal by the things which we suffer."

Steven Cramer offers these words of hope and wisdom: "Someday, on the other side of eternity, we will be able to look back over life's adversities [even those brought on us by other people hurting us]—and we will be able to see divine purpose in them as they gave us experience, built character, and helped us learn how much we needed the Savior in our daily lives. . . .

"You can test this principle of divine purpose in adversity by tracing the pattern of your own experience. Examine a situation in your life which now brings you great joy. Trace it back through the genealogy of circumstance that preceded the present victory, and you will inevitably find that its roots lie in some challenge of the past, some weakness or difficulty which once gave you great sorrow."

"And we know that *all* things work together for good to them that love God" (Rom. 8:28, emphasis added).

Joseph's Struggle to Forgive

Even Joseph, son of Jacob, did not find forgiveness easy, but his suffering ultimately brought about a great blessing. Wendy Ulrich offers a very interesting perspective: "[Joseph was] sold into slavery in Egypt by his ten older brothers. Surely this is not a trivial trespass, but a major, atrocious offense. After trapping Joseph (apparently still a boy) in a pit used to ensnare animals, the brothers taunt Joseph, threatening to murder him. When they decide against murder, Judah, one of the brothers, proposes selling him to a passing caravan as a slave. Against his pleas and terrified cries, Joseph's brothers turn deaf ears, sending him to an unknown, potentially torturous fate. The heinousness of their crime against Joseph is undeniable.

"Also undeniable is Joseph's favor with God, and his personal righteousness in the face of considerable obstacles. He is blessed by God with spiritual gifts, influential friends, and political opportunity. Yet, even honorable Joseph does not deal easily with his painful past. His anger, hurt, and lonely suffering are almost tangible years later when he names his son Manasseh, which, he tells us, signifies that the Lord has caused him to forget all his toil and all in his father's house. He names his second son Ephraim, signifying that God had made him fruitful in the land of his afflictions. We can feel the pain and sorrow implicit in these statements. Even when he has the resources and power, he makes no known attempt to contact his family. To the contrary, he makes every effort to maintain distance, ignore his family, and forget his pain.

". . . Because of Joseph's influence, Egypt prepares for the predicted famine, [and] Joseph's brothers . . . journey to Egypt, bowing to their unrecognized brother as they ask to purchase grain. . . . [Joseph's] conflicting emotions are apparent as he flees to his chamber to weep, perhaps remembering the hatred of his brothers, the forsaken panic of being sold by his own siblings, the terrors of his early years in slavery. . . .

". . . Forgiveness does not come easily to Joseph—despite his righteousness, his years of distance from the original offense, his maturity, and his favor with God. He even repeats the sin of his offenders . . . setting up a situation that would result in his beloved younger brother enduring the same anguish of threatened separation from family. . . . He, of all people, should have known the terror such an act might inflict. . . .

"The brothers do not abandon Benjamin [as they had done Joseph] but return to plead for his life. Judah, the very brother who thought of selling Joseph, steps forward and . . . pleads with Joseph to accept him as a slave in Benjamin's place, as his father would surely die of grief if he were to lose his last born.

"As Joseph witnesses his greatest offender offer his life,

showing his true repentance, Joseph's heart is deeply touched. At long last he sends his servants out, weeping openly as he reveals his identity to his incredulous family. . . . At this moment, Joseph receives the inspired understanding that God used his enslavement both to empower Joseph and to save his father's house from starvation. Joseph sees the blessings that have come to him and to his family despite the sins committed—evidence of God's great mercy for them all.

"There is an interesting footnote to this story. When Jacob was on his deathbed, he requested that his sons ask Joseph, in his behalf, to forgive them. This is the first incidence of the word 'forgive' in the Bible (Genesis 50:17). . . . Joseph sets vengeance aside, he comforts his brothers, and deals kindly with them. He reminds his brothers that even though their intentions had been evil (Joseph does not vacillate on this point of justice), God had worked these things for the good of all" ("When Forgiveness Flounders," *Spiritual Recovery*, 349–352).

Gratitude for Lessons Learned

We are told that there are four stages of recovery and healing from any loss:

1- Shock/Denial
2- Awareness/ Blaming
3- Growth/Acceptance
4- Gratitude

Our hypothetical situation from the previous chapter will

illustrate these four stages. You have driven into the crowded parking lot of a busy store. You are glad to see a parking space being vacated near the entrance to the store and position your car to take the spot as soon as the other car is out of the way. You even have your signal light on.

But, before you can take action, another vehicle whips around the corner and zips into that spot before you have a chance to move.

Your first reaction is *shock/denial*: "I can't believe he took my space!"

Second comes *awareness/blaming*: "I have just been trespassed against. What a jerk!"

The third step is *growth/acceptance*: "Oh well, those things happen. I'll have to find another parking place, albeit farther away from the door." It is likely you will have forgotten the incident by the time you enter the store.

The final stage is *gratitude*. Gratitude? Yes, gratitude.

In this situation, you could be grateful that it was necessary for you to find a parking spot further from the store, for it gave you the opportunity of walking—and we all know how important exercise is.

For all you know, the difference in timing might actually have been a protective blessing to you, preventing you from being hit by a truck later on. You should thank that person who delayed you!

At the very least, you can be grateful that the experience gave you a heightened awareness of how it feels to have such a thing happen. In the future you will, with your increased sensitivity, be certain that you never do such a thing to anyone else.

Through the anguish of adversity we can learn and we can grow. And when we are able to look back on painful events and feel a sense of gratitude for the things we learned and the growth we experienced—then we know that we have forgiven and our healing is complete. We have allowed those experiences to become our best teachers.

Surrendering

"Actually, it is our own stubbornness that determines how difficult our lessons have to be. Jesus Christ loves us enough to do whatever it takes, no matter how tough it gets, to win our loyalty and devotion and to cleanse our lives of the things that keep us from his fellowship. If we resist the lessons he provides, if we rebel and refuse to learn, the afflictions will be repeated over and over, with greater and greater intensity, until we finally humble ourselves and learn what we need to change" (Steven Cramer, *In the Arms of His Love*).

Wayne Dyer agrees: "I can assure you that once you no longer need the lessons in your life that unpleasant events offer you, you will no longer have these events. If forgiveness is something you need to practice, you will continue to attract opportunities to practice it."

Blessings in Disguise

In recalling my own painful journey, I feel gratitude now for the changes it brought into my life. The situation forced me to look at myself, and I didn't like what I saw. I had great need for change—to become less judgmental and more compassionate and sensitive toward others. Wayne Dyer spoke the truth when he said, "Everything that happened to you is a lesson you can be grateful for."

I thought of the things I had learned and the growth experienced through my own struggle, recounting some of the blessings that had come as a result of this pain-filled experience.

First, when my own family turned away, I was compelled to turn to my Father in Heaven and the Savior, compelled to seek and find a closer relationship with them rather than leaning on my family for my security, my strength, and my sense of self-worth.

Second, it made my new husband Micheal and my new-found, budding relationship strong from the beginning, as we stood together alone. He offered me unconditional love and acceptance and his full support and sympathy, even while he allowed me to experience my pain and to seek and struggle for my own answers.

Third, it has helped me to appreciate my mother more than ever, as she was the only family member unable to abide by the family edict to ostracize me (my father is deceased). She has endeared herself to me even more by demonstrating her unfailing love.

Fourth, in going through all this, I have hungered deeply to learn. And even as I have learned, Heavenly Father has blessed me with opportunities to share with others the things I have learned. Helping others who also may be struggling has been one of the greatest joys of my life.

Without the negative things I experienced, I would not have been so motivated to learn nor so deeply committed in my heart to what I now believe to be the true Gospel of Jesus Christ. Rather than mere rigid obedience to rules, it is a gospel of love for one another. It includes a respect for agency, a consideration for relationships, and a willingness to love even "sinners," as Christ did. It is being filled with charity and forgiveness for one's self and for others. In the depths of my soul, I learned that "he that loveth not, knoweth not God, for God is love." For this knowledge, for this conversion to the true Gospel of Jesus Christ, I will be eternally grateful. Thus, I could dedicate this book "to my family members, who were my best teachers."

Finally, I cannot help but believe in my heart that the blessing of being able to give birth after a lifetime of infertility has been a tangible reminder of Heavenly Father's compensation for my other losses. Not only was my first "homemade" baby born when I was 41, but, incredibly, at the age of 44, I gave birth to a second miracle baby born on the 25th of July 1995! Our baby has been named Hunter, in honor of Howard W. Hunter, whose statement came at a time in my life when I so much needed to be reassured of the essence of the Gospel: "I would invite all . . . to live with ever more attention to the life and example of the Lord Jesus Christ, especially the love and hope and compassion He displayed. I pray that we might treat each other with more kindness, more courtesy, more humility and patience and forgiveness."

CHAPTER THIRTEEN

Forgiving Yourself

*He has borne the awful burden
so we can be gentle with ourselves.*
—UNKNOWN

FOR YEARS TOM Anderson's life was blighted by the memory of his part in a fraternity escapade that resulted in the death of one of his classmates. He floundered from one job to another. He and Betty, his wife, separated after six years of marriage. Then something changed. His wife came back; he earned a good position. What had changed his life?

He explained, "I used to think, 'Nothing can undo what I have done.' The thought of my guilt would stop me in the middle of a smile or a handshake. It put a wall between Betty and me. Then I had an unexpected visit from the person I dreaded most to see—the mother of the college classmate who had died."

Her message was simple. "'Years ago, I found it in my heart, through prayer, to forgive you. Betty forgave you. So did your friends and employers." She paused, and then said sternly, "You are the one person who hasn't forgiven Tom Anderson. Who do you think you are to stand out against the people of this town and the Lord Almighty?"

"I looked into her eyes and found there a kind of permission to be the person I might have been if her boy had lived. For the first time in my adult life I felt worthy to love and be loved."

Our peace and progress depend upon forgiving not only others, but ourselves, as well. You may ask, "But doesn't my continued remorse and internal suffering for wrongs I have committed prove how sorry I am, demonstrating that I am willing to pay the uttermost farthing?" Perhaps this convoluted thinking is exactly what Satan would want for us. Discouragement is one of his best tools. Additionally, we shall see that forgiving others comes as a result of being able to forgive ourselves first.

"Love Thy Neighbor as Thyself"

The remarkable truth is that we really do love our neighbor as we love ourselves. We cannot love others if we are full of self-loathing. We may go through the motions of forgiving others, but it may not be real or lasting. As my friend observed, "If you have not forgiven yourself, the forgiveness you think you've extended to others is half-baked."

Wayne Dyer said, "Once you accept yourself completely, you will know when you have mastered the art of self-forgiveness. When you are no longer judgmental toward others, you will have forgiven yourself and be on your path [to peace and happiness]. Releasing judgment of another is actually releasing judgment of yourself. . . . When you stop doing this, you have for-given yourself for whatever aspect of yourself you see in them. . . . Self-acceptance will turn into self-love, and when you are filled with self-love, that is what you will have to give away."

Loving and forgiving starts with yourself.

"Thou Doest the Same Things"

Isn't it queer that we dislike most in others those unpleasant characteristics we possess ourselves? Using a personal example, I like to think of myself as being very thrifty, prudent, and frugal when it comes to spending money. I will go to great lengths to save a few dimes. At garage sales I have been known to talk the seller down further from the low price he was asking in the first place. Yet, I hate it when others are that way with me! I think of them as stingy, miserly, cheap, penny-pinching tightwads and skinflints! I must admit that, in truth, I really don't like that wretched part of me—thus my difficulty in tolerating it in others.

Truly, we see and condemn our own weaknesses in others. One wrote, "It has become clear to me that the real reason for all the hurt feelings we experience is that we are defending what we cannot forgive in ourselves."

Paul said: "Thou art inexcusable, O man, whosoever thou art that judgest: for wherein thou judgest another, thou con-demnest thyself; for *thou that judgest doest the same things*" (Rom. 2:1; emphasis added).

God Doesn't Grade on the Curve!

One woman was asked why she had given up going to church as a teenager. She replied, "I remember sitting in my youth class, and the teacher was telling us how good and how pure we had to be to go to heaven. She taught us how hard it would be to repent if we made a mistake, and that even if we did repent we could never have the same blessings as before. Of course, by then I had already made my mistakes.

"Then she made a point of telling us that only a special few could find the strait and narrow way, and when I looked around that room and saw my competition, all of those goody-goodies, I knew I didn't have a snowball's chance of being one of the few, so I just gave up and quit going."

When asked why she had returned after more than a decade, she answered, "At first all I knew was that I had to get out of the dark, but as I moved closer and closer to the light, I finally realized that my teacher hadn't told the truth. There is room for me in the kingdom of God, and I don't have to compete with the goody-goodies to get there. I'm not competing with anyone but myself. I have repented, I've already found the strait and narrow way, and as long as I'm just a little better this month than I was last month, just a little nicer, a little kinder, a little more compassionate—in his name and for his sake—then I win it all."

This woman realized that God has provided a way for *all* of His children to return to Him. She accepted Christ's atonement by repenting and by forgiving herself.

Forgiving our shortcomings doesn't mean denying that they exist. On the contrary, it means facing them honestly, realistically.

Guilt is a smoke alarm, a warning signal that we have transgressed and need to correct our course. We must listen to the warning voice of guilt and react promptly through repentance. Otherwise, guilt becomes shame—toxic shame. Satan then has his day, influencing us to believe that we are unworthy, beyond redemption, that it is too late, our sins too deep.

It is through repentance and forgiveness of our mistakes that we gain freedom to learn from experience. Then we can move forward in our lives.

Learning from Life's Lessons

I have read or heard numerous accounts of near-death experiences. For some, their life reviews were very distressing as they experienced the pain that they had caused others during their lives. Still, they felt the Being of Light helping them through their life reviews, all the while radiating pure love, understanding, and compassion, his message to them being, "You were just learning."

This concept was reinforced in one particular account, as the woman shared the insights she had gained before returning to life. "Forgiveness of ourselves is where all forgiveness starts, because we can't love others if we don't first love ourselves, and if we are to overcome the hardships that we will inevitably face, we must accept all of our experiences as good, however bad they seem, for they help us in the spiritual growth we are here on earth to accomplish.

"God is the judge of each of our lives, and only he really knows the depth of each soul's trials. We are here to learn, to experience life by using our free will. You can still use your free will to change your heart, forgive yourself, and move back to God. You have made mistakes, but you can still feel his love.

"They don't see sin in the spirit world as we do. God knew we would make mistakes. Life is all about mistakes. It is constant change and growth. Our greatest challenges in life will one day be known to us as our greatest teacher" (Betty J. Eadie, *The Awakening Heart* [1996], 118).

If God is patient with us, then surely we can be gentle with ourselves. God loves each of us, no matter where we are. We judge ourselves and thus keep ourselves from God, not the other way around.

How do you treat yourself when you make mistakes? Do you tell yourself that you are a bad person—or do you consider yourself to be a good person who makes mistakes? You were doing the best you knew how at the time.

One woman wrote me: "I am now more at peace with myself. I have had the hardest time forgiving myself for what I perceived as mistakes when actually they were learning experiences. I forgive myself and [my former husband]—we just did not have the knowledge to survive all the things we went through."

None of us are free of flaws. Wisdom lies in the gift of forgiving our human failings—to tumble, pick ourselves up, shake the dust off our spirits, and try to avoid the next mistake. We all yearn to be decent people.

Neal A. Maxwell stated: "He who was thrust down delights in having us put ourselves down. Self-contempt is of Satan; there is none of it in heaven. We should, of course, learn from our mistakes, but without reviewing the instant replays lest these become the game of life itself. . . ."

It is difficult for me to envision a heaven where people are wandering around with furrowed brows and slumping shoulders mumbling, "I shouldn't be here. I don't deserve to be here. I made mistakes. I'm not good enough."

"God, our Father, has a perfect faith in each of us. . . . By allowing us to choose between spiritual life and death and by giving us the means to repent and to be forgiven, He has already given us the assurance that we can return to Him. He has expressed a perfect belief in our ability to succeed while here on earth by virtue of His sending us here.

"Although we may get discouraged from time to time and—if only for a moment—believe that we cannot change or improve, we must quickly separate ourselves from our failure and remember that failure is an *event*, never a *person*. God did not make any failures. Instead, He created changing, growing, developing sons and daughters who can become like Him.

"This precious perspective will strengthen our hope as life's lessons refine and define us" (Lloyd Newell, *The Divine Connection*, 213, 259).

The past is over, and everything you did got you where you are at this moment. Everything happened exactly as it did in order for you to learn the lessons you needed to learn. You needed to do it all. Now lovingly forgive yourself. Receive the lesson from it. The more willing you are to be gentle with yourself, the more you will find forgiveness a way of life.

"This Means You!"

One woman wrote: "When I was a little girl, my teenage brother posted a notice on the door to his bedroom. It said simply: KEEP OUT! THIS MEANS YOU!

"I thought how interesting that he would say that. His room was in the basement, and when cousins came or friends were here, they rarely went down to the basement. . . . Meanwhile, I blissfully went in and out of his room whenever I wanted to.

"It wasn't until years later, after my brother had gone off to college, that I reread that notice still on his door—and finally realized that the message had really been meant for me!"

If the ability to forgive others is a desirable quality, then why do we not think it desirable to forgive ourselves? If judging others is something we know we ought to avoid, then why do we not avoid judging ourselves? If blame is damaging and destructive, then why do we feel a need to continue to blame ourselves? If harboring up resentments toward others is an obstacle to our own spiritual progress, then what compels us to harbor up such feelings against ourselves? Do not the gospel concepts of love and mercy, compassion and kindness apply to ourselves as well as to others?

You have not fully accepted the Atonement of Jesus Christ until you realize that it reaches all men, including yourself. The Lord said, "of you it is required to forgive all men" (D&C 64:10). This means you!

God's Power and Mercy

Gordon B. Hinckley stated, "There is a mighty power of healing in Christ, and . . . if we are to be his true servants, we must not only exercise that healing power in behalf of others, but, perhaps more importantly, inwardly."

I must recognize that God is both powerful and merciful enough to forgive even my sins. As one recalled, "I knew about God, but I didn't know God. As I came to know the Lord, I learned to know His nature, to feel His mercy that surpasses justice."

"For I am able to make you holy, and your sins are forgiven you" (D&C 60:7).

Mercy cannot rob justice, but through the Savior's Atonement mercy can satisfy the demands of justice and will triumph in the end. We must exercise mercy toward ourselves and others.

Our Father in Heaven is "a God ready to pardon, gracious and merciful, slow to anger, and of great kindness" (Neh. 9:17).

"For I will be merciful to their unrighteousness, and their sins and their iniquities will I remember no more" (Heb. 8:12). When God declares He will remember our sins no more, perhaps He is inviting us to do the same. It causes me to realize that He probably has better things to do than dwell on our past mistakes. And so do we. The past is to learn from, not to live in. Let's get on with life!

Self Judgement

As children of Christ, we feel love and forgiveness;
Compassion through Christ's great atonement for sin.
We comprehend mercy and understand weakness
And give up self-judgment through following Him.
—KATHLEEN SOUTHARD

One woman said to me, "I realized that failure to forgive myself was actually the failure to acknowledge and accept the Savior's atonement."

Another added her insight. "The atonement has shown me that I am worth the Savior's precious life. How then can I refuse to accept his evaluation of me? To do so would be to declare myself a better judge of myself than He is!"

We must give up our pride — or, rather, our *reverse* pride. When we fail to forgive ourselves, it is as though we are asserting, "My power to do wrong is greater than God's power to make right. My power to mess up is greater than God's power to repair and redeem and restore. I, with all my foolishness and folly, am greater than Christ with all His mercy and His love. My sins are too complex for even God to resolve!"

Though feelings of remorse may begin the process of repentance, we needn't continue to "beat ourselves up" or to dwell on our past mistakes. Richard L. Evans said: "Life moves in one direction only—and each day we are faced with an actual set of circumstances, not with what might have been, not with what we might have done, but with what *is,* and with where we are *now*— and from this point we must proceed: not from where we were, not from where we wish we were—but from where we *are.*

"What we cannot change should not needlessly keep us from looking and moving forward. Nothing lost or left behind should keep us from becoming what we can become, from learning what we can learn. . . .

"Whatever the past or its meaning, or its length or its losses, or its lessons learned or left unlearned, we go on from where we are—wherever it is—and become what we can become; with work, repentance, improvement; with faith in the future."

Christ suffered *for us* if we would repent. *He* paid the price so that we need no longer suffer. Let not his sacrifice for me and for you have been in vain.

"Behold, he who has repented of his sins, the same is forgiven, and I the Lord, remember them no more" (D&C 58:42). We can do likewise.

CHAPTER FOURTEEN

To Be Like the Savior

*I have felt that the ultimate form of love
for God and men is forgiveness.*

—MARION D. HANKS

I HAVE LEARNED that if our lives and faith are centered on Jesus Christ—if we come unto him—nothing can ever go permanently wrong. Nothing can hurt us if we can feel his love for us, recognizing that he has offered to take our burdens on himself.

Christ said of himself: "The Spirit of the Lord is upon me, because he hath anointed me to preach the gospel to the poor, he hath sent me to heal the brokenhearted, to preach deliverance to the captives, and recovering of sight to the blind, to set at liberty them that are bruised" (Luke 4:18). Surely those of us who are imprisoned by past hurts, unable to forgive ourselves or others, fit these descriptions.

Trusting God

God is anxious to comfort and to bless when we are finally humble enough to ask Him with a sincere heart. Indeed, prayer is not conquering God's reluctance, but taking hold of God's willingness. Yet, He can only mend a broken heart if we are willing to give Him all the pieces.

Sometimes our petitions may seem to go unanswered. There may be lessons we need to learn before our request for relief is granted, however fervently we may plead. We must trust God—trust His timing as well as His power. Then we can be comforted in knowing that God gives the very best to those who leave the choice to Him. God may not come when you want Him to, but He will always be on time. When we "let go and let God" and trust Him enough to be willing to forgive as He has asked us to, we can be assured that He will heal the hurts of our hearts.

When we forgive, we are made whole. As we faithfully surrender to the Savior our pain caused by others, the power of the Atonement heals our wounded hearts, lifts our burdens of sorrow, and brings peace to our souls.

"I have heard thy prayer, I have seen thy tears: behold, I will heal thee" (2 Kings 20:5).

"Come unto me, all ye that labor and are heavy laden, and I will give you rest" (Matt. 11:22).

"The gospel of Christ brings the peace of God, which passeth all understanding" (Philip. 4:7).

Paul defines how we should act in the face of trouble from an adversary. Call it charity, call it compassion, call it love or mercy—it is what enables us to meet opposition and frustration. Paul says to bear all things and to endure all things. He says charity suffereth long and is kind. That is the pathway to Christ.

The Comforting Message of the Atonement

The Savior is our model of forgiveness who, even as He suffered torture and death, petitioned God in behalf of the soldiers, entreating, "Father, forgive them; for they know not what they do" (Luke 23:34).

We may not deserve our suffering—but neither did Christ deserve to be crucified.

Wendy Ulrich connected forgiveness with our willingness to follow the Savior when she said, "Christ voluntarily endured and experienced through the Atonement the full range of every agony, every struggle, distress, torment, grief, suffering, pain, and hurt we undergo. If he is willing to forgive, having been sin's victim beyond mortal ability to endure, then he can rightfully ask us to forgive also. As we feel with him, in our hearts we long to [be like him and to] forgive as he directs."

Harboring hurts by others can canker our souls, preventing us from experiencing the full blessings of the Atonement. It takes true faith in the Lord to submit offenses against us to the power of Christ's atonement.

Let us cultivate that aspect of our character and rejoice in the spirit of forgiveness which is the comforting message of the Atonement. Let us think of the Atonement—how all-encompassing is its forgiveness. When you can genuinely forgive and move on, then you have taken upon yourself His name. You have become a true follower of Christ. Would you be close to the Lord? Forgiving others is the price.

The Forgiving Heart

The Apostle Paul wrote to the Saints in Ephesus, "And be ye kind one to another, tender-hearted, forgiving one another, even as God for Christ's sake hath forgiven you" (Eph. 4:32).

As a friend explained, "Forgiveness is an act of faith in the beginning, and an act of charity in the end. We do it because Heavenly Father tells us it is the healthy thing to do. But every time we choose it, it becomes more a part of our nature, and we become more charitable as it is incorporated into our characters."

Forgive? Will I forgive, you cry.
But what is the gift, the favor?
You would lift me from my poor place
To stand beside the Savior.
You would have me see with His eyes, smile,
And with Him reach out to salve a sorrowing heart—
For one small moment to share in Christ's great art.
Will I forgive, you cry. Oh, may I—may I?
—CAROL LYNN PEARSON, "*The Forgiving*"

"We need to be kinder with one another, more gentle and more forgiving. we need to be slower to anger and more prompt to help. We need to extend the hand of friendship and resist the hand of retribution. In short, we need to love one another with the pure love of Christ, with genuine charity and compassion," urged Howard W. Hunter.

If our goal here in mortality is to attain the qualities of godhood, to become like God, then we *must* learn to forgive as He does.

It is a happy person who remembers kindness and forgets offenses. It is far more noble to conquer one's own dark passion than to crush a foe; and sweeter than revenge are his feelings who, when his enemy hungers, feeds him; when he thirsts, gives him drink. In so doing, man experiences somewhat of the nature and tastes something of the happiness of God.

When the Savior counseled his followers to forgive "seventy times seven" it was as though he was instructing them that, rather than forgiveness consisting of singular responses to isolated incidents, it should be a way of life, a state of the heart.

Roderick J. Linton, in his article, "The Forgiving Heart: Changing the Way We Look at Life," addressed this concept. "Forgiveness is a personal attribute, not just a decision we make from time to time when we feel we should. To have a forgiving heart is to see the world in a different light. It is to forsake the tendency to judge, condemn, exclude, or hate any human soul. A forgiving heart seeks to love and to be patient with imperfection. The forgiving heart understands that we are all in need of the atonement of Jesus Christ.

"A forgiving heart is one of the most Christlike virtues we can possess. If we have a forgiving heart, our very nature will be kind, patient, long-suffering, and charitable. Forgiveness plants and nourishes the seeds of Christlike love in both the giver and the receiver. Indeed, forgiveness, in its fullest expression, is synonymous with charity, the pure love of Christ.

"Those who reject the forgiving heart and choose instead to

harbor resentments, bitterness, and revenge, see the world through darkened glasses. They are quick to take offense, always assuming the worst in others' motives. They feel the pain of human relationships more intensely. They are intolerant of the differences that exist between themselves and others. Such persons tend to be lonely because they can find no one to meet their standard. They are often angry with themselves because they are no more forgiving of their own faults than they are of the faults of others. . . . Joy finds no place in their hearts" (*Ensign*, Apr. 1993, 15).

We may lash out at another, feeling justified in our feelings of revenge and lack of love. In these moments we have forgotten the message and example of the Savior. We have much need for forgiveness, much need to be forgiven. Only then can we heal or be healed.

Even As He Walked

John tells us: "And hereby we do know that we know him, if we keep his commandments. He that saith, I know him, and keepeth not his commandments, is a liar, and the truth is not in him. But whoso keepeth his word, in him verily is the love of God perfected: hereby know we that we are in him. He that saith he abideth in him ought himself also so to walk, even as he walked" (I John 2:3-6).

"If a man say, I love God, and hateth his brother, he is a liar: for he that loveth not his brother whom he hath seen, how can he love God whom he hath not seen" (I John 4:20)?

"Again, a new commandment I write unto you, which thing is true in him and in you: because the darkness is past, and the true light now shineth. He that saith he is in the light and hateth his brother, is in darkness even until now. He that loveth his brother abideth in the light, and there is none occasion of stumbling in him. But he that hateth his brother is in darkness, and walketh in darkness, and knoweth not whither he goeth, because that darkness hath blinded his eyes" (I John 2:8-11).

Christ said, "Inasmuch as ye have done it unto one of the least of these my brethren, ye have done it unto me" (Matt. 25:40). Who does the "least of these" refer to? The poor and the needy? The sick and the afflicted? Children? Perhaps all of these. But *in the eternal perspective, "the least" are sinners*, those who break commandments, as defined by Christ in Matthew 5:19. Yet, the Savior said that the way I treat that sinner—or that person who has sinned against me—is the same as treating Him that way.

He forgave sinners, even as he hung on a cross fashioned by them. Not only did he forgive them, but he asked his Father to forgive them. We can do the same. "He that saith he abideth in him ought himself also to walk, even as he walked."

On the other hand, ". . . the withholding of love is the negation of the spirit of Christ, the proof that we never knew him, that for us he lived in vain. It means that he suggested nothing in all our thoughts, that he inspired nothing in all our lives, that we were not once near enough to him to be seized with the spell of his compassion for the world."

The grace of God is sufficient to overcome sins of every kind—except having a hard heart and a proud spirit. If we are honest, we must acknowledge that a hard heart and a proud spirit are what we possess when we are not willing to let go and forgive.

"Forgive our sins as we forgive,"
Thou taught us, Lord, to pray;
But thou alone can grant us grace
To live the words we say.

How can pardon reach and bless
The unforgiving heart
That broods on wrongs and will not let
Old bitterness depart?

In blazing light your cross reveals
The truth we dimly knew:
What trivial debts are owed to us,
How great our debt to you!

Lord, cleanse the depths within our souls,
And bid resentment cease;
Then, bound to all in bonds of love,
Our lives will spread thy peace.
—ROSAMOND E. HERKLOTS

CHAPTER FIFTEEN

Pride: The Great Obstacle to Our Forgiving

The proud are easily offended and hold grudges.
They withold forgiveness to justify their injured feelings.

—EZRA TAFT BENSON

EAVENLY FATHER HAD been so patient and so good to me on my journey to forgiveness, allowing me to learn at my own pace, a step at a time, as I was ready. I thought I "had it all together."

The manuscript for the earlier edition of this book was at the press waiting to be printed. It was time to do another radio program, the ninth on the subject of forgiveness. But in the night, I experienced a stupor of thought regarding the subject I'd intended to address. Instead, I was led to understand that I should speak on pride.

I felt uncomfortable with the subject; perhaps it hit "too close to home." It seemed that, in order for me to admit that I had a problem with pride, I would have to be gut-wrenchingly honest and totally humble—the very opposite of being proud! Pride: so easy to recognize in others, yet difficult to admit in ourselves. But perhaps it is one of the greatest obstacles to our ability to forgive others and, ultimately, our passageway into the Kingdom of God.

As I recalled my own struggle and my earlier beliefs about forgiveness (see Chapter 1), I was interested now to observe that my beliefs were laced with an underlying pride.

The Author of Pride

Who is the author of pride and selfishness? What is the first example that we find of it in the scriptures? In Moses we read of a council in heaven before the world was. ". . . Satan . . . came before me saying—Behold, here am *I*, send *me*, *I* will be thy son, and *I* will redeem all mankind, that one soul shall not be lost, and surely *I* will do it; wherefore, give *me* thine honor" (Moses 4:1; emphasis added). It is interesting to note that within five short lines of scripture, Satan refers to himself six times.

Christ, in contrast, said, "Father, *thy* will be done, and the glory be *thine* forever."

Satan rebelled and was cast down "And he became Satan, yea, even the devil, the father of all lies, to deceive and to blind men, and to lead them captive at his will" (Moses 4:4). Just as Lucifer was and is filled with pride and anger, so now he uses those characteristics to ensnare us today, even to deceive those who consider themselves most righteous.

C. Terry Warner spoke of "Lucifer's method of waging the Great War he began in heaven against his own brothers and sisters. He had proposed a scheme that he maintained would benefit us all, but was really for his own glory. So when his self-nom-ination was rejected, he smarted with disappointment and resentment, and set out to make anyone and everyone pay for his defeat. Unwilling, like many of us, to take responsibility for his sin, he sought to shift it elsewhere. . . . He spread his discontent to throngs of others, stoked their indignation, and marshaled them into a coalition sustained by their shared resentment. In just this pattern, . . . first [there is] conflict within ourselves over our own failure to be as we ought to be—honest, simple, solid, and true—and then the inevitable diminishment or manipula-tion of others. . . . Whether it draws blood or wears a civil face, strife among us divides us, takes away our spiritual breath, sweeps us into spirals of retaliation and misery, and gradually addicts us to resentment and revenge" ("Honest, Simple, Solid, True," *Brigham Young Magazine*, June 1996, 32–39).

Satan uses pride to "deceive and blind" us. When we are not able to forgive another, do we not consider ourselves the inno-cent victim, therefore believing ourselves to be morally superior to that person who has wronged us? In our self-righteousness, are we not saying that he does not deserve our forgiveness or our love? That we have the right to judge him as to whether or not he is worthy of our forgiveness? Do we believe that our forgiving him would be acquiescence, giving in, backing down, an admis-sion that we were wrong? And do not all these attitudes reek with pride?

The Universal Sin

Ezra Taft Benson delivered a powerful address on the subject of pride. I have taken the liberty of extracting the portions of
his talk that deal specifically with the state of the heart that prevents us from being able to forgive.

"Most of us think of pride as self-centeredness, conceit,
boastfulness, arrogance, or haughtiness. All of these are elements
of the sin, but the heart, or core, is still missing. The center fea-
ture of pride is enmity—enmity toward God and enmity toward
our fellowmen. *Enmity* means "hatred toward, hostility to, or a
state of opposition." It is the power by which Satan wishes to
reign over us.

"Pride is a sin that can readily be seen in others but is rarely
admitted in ourselves. Most of us consider pride to be a sin of
those on the top, such as the rich and the learned, looking down
at the rest of us. There is, however, a far more common ailment
among us—and that is from the bottom looking up. It is mani-
fest in so many ways, such as fault-finding, gossiping, backbiting,
murmuring . . . and being unforgiving. . . .

"Selfishness is one of the more common faces of pride.
'How everything affects me' is the center of all that matters—"
He mentions self-pity. Isn't this what we feel when we choose to
take offense and feel hurt?

"Another face of pride is contention. . . . The scriptures tell
us that 'only by pride cometh contention' (Proverbs 13:10).

"The scriptures testify that the proud are easily offended
and hold grudges. They withhold forgiveness to keep another in
their debt and to justify their injured feelings. . . . Defensiveness

is used by them to justify and rationalize their frailties and failures.

"Pride is a damning sin in the true sense of that word. It limits or stops [our own] progression. The proud are not easily taught. They won't change their minds to accept truths, because to do so implies they have been wrong.

"Pride adversely affects all our relationships. . . . Our degree of pride determines how we treat our God and our brothers and sisters.

"We must cleanse the inner vessel by conquering pride. Pride affects all of us at various times and in various degrees. Pride is the universal sin, the great vice.

"The antidote for pride is humility, meekness, submissiveness. It is the broken heart and contrite spirit.

"God will have a humble people. . . . We can choose to be humble ourselves by forgiving those who have offended us. . . . Let us choose to be humble. We can do it. I know we can" (*Ensign*, May 1989, 4–7).

A Meek and Quiet Spirit

David O. McKay stated, "Humility is the solid foundation of all the virtues." We know that it is an essential ingredient of charity (see I Cor. 13:4–6). A careful search of the scriptures will show that the Lord "resisteth the proud, and giveth grace to the humble" (I Pet. 5:5). A quick review of various concordances under the key word *humility* and its synonyms (humble, penitent, meek, contrite, mild, submissive, etc.) will reveal many more scriptures extolling humility before God.

Christ demonstrated that meek spirit which is the antithesis of pride. He is our example, as he said in Matthew 11:29: ". . . Learn of me; for I am meek and lowly in heart." He personifies that meekness by the way in which he deals with us.

Malcolm Muggeridge related love of God to the washing of the disciples' feet. "Jesus demonstrated once and for all that the Son of Man was the servant of man; that whatsoever was arrogant, assertive, dogmatic, or demagogic belonged to the gospel of power, not to his gospel of love . . . that in abasing themselves, men attain the highest heights, and in glorifying themselves, they sink to the lowest depths" (*Jesus, the Man Who Lives*, 151–152).

Speaking of the Lord, C. Terry Warner said: "He stands before me as One who absolutely does not oppose me. He does not compete with me when I want to take things for my selfish purposes. He has no interest whatsoever in dominating me. He does not resist my injustice. If I hurt him by offending his children, he takes no vengeance. He is vulnerable, meek, and lowly of heart. This meekness works upon me as no other influence can. It is the one influence that is unfailingly capable of making me ashamed of my insensitivity and injustice; it calls upon me to question how I have used my freedom. His willingness to suffer at my hand, if I choose to abuse him, robs me of the rationalizations I have constructed to justify myself.

"If others defend themselves against my insensitivity or unfairness, I feel accused, treated violently. I can then [justify myself by saying], 'They deserve this treatment: just look at how insensitively (or unfairly) they are treating me.'

"The Savior by contrast does not resist my evil and thereby heaps coals of fire—coals of shame and remorse and hot repentance—upon my head. I am humbled in the only way a person can be humbled—that is, in the face of humility" ("Peace First, Then Order," BYU Women's Week, Apr. 1990).

Sometimes we think of meekness as being spineless. Not so. Meekness simply means submitting one's will to the will of the Father. Sometimes that calls for action, as when Christ cleansed the temple. Sometimes it calls for longsuffering.

Charity is defined specifically in 1 Corinthians 13. This scripture also defines what charity is not. "Charity vaunteth not herself . . . is not puffed up . . . seeketh not her own. . . ." Are these not perfect descriptions of pride and selfishness, the very opposite of charity?

It takes a great deal of courage to face oneself honestly and to admit that it is pride, the "great vice, the universal sin," that is preventing our forgiving and damning our progress.

It is no wonder that, in order to qualify for the Kingdom of God, we are admonished to become as little children, who are characterized as being "submissive, meek, humble, patient, full of love . . ."—qualities that are totally foreign to one with a proud, unforgiving heart.

As I spoke about pride during that radio show—and in the days that followed— my own feelings of discomfort grew. I had thought that I had this forgiveness business figured out. I felt like an authority on the subject. (Does not being an *author* make one an *authority?*) I became increasingly aware, however, that the Lord wasn't finished with me yet. He had only been letting me take a rest, a time out, before compelling me to move onward and upward to the next level and to face the most difficult thing of all—myself.

CHAPTER SIXTEEN

The Rest of the Journey

Satan does not need to overpower
us in order to win the war.
He only needs to get us to
adopt his way of fighting it.

—C. TERRY WARNER

A
T ALMOST THE same time as my encounter
with the subject of pride, I was able to hear an
address by C. Terry Warner, a man whose ideas I had already
come to respect. I was in the middle of baking bread when the
speech was broadcast, so we videotaped it to hear it later. Again
and again I listened to it, the painful unrest inside me growing
greater each time. My husband tried to cheer me. "You are on the
verge of making another breakthrough," he said. Even in my
misery, I also sensed something significant about to happen.

"If You Had Come unto Me . . ."

Perhaps the part of his talk that struck me with the greatest
force was the account of the woman who felt herself the victim
of her husband's emotional neglect. "When she tried to talk
about why he was distant, he said it was because she was always

angry. This angered her more, and she told him she was only angry because of his lack of love, which made him more inclined to withdraw. . . . She went to the mountains alone, intent upon reading one of the contemporary self-help books. She wrote later:

"'As the writer began describing the intense need we each have for love, I began to feel more and more deprived, until I felt such a huge longing that I could barely breathe. I decided to write all of this down for my husband to read, and enumerate the many times I had felt emotionally deprived. I began to write furiously, to pour it all out onto the paper. The longer I wrote, the more I began to have a feeling come over me that what I was writing was false. The feeling continued growing until I could no longer squelch it, and I knew intuitively that the feeling was coming from God, that He was telling me that what I was writing was false. "How could it be false?" I asked angrily. "I lived it. I know it was there because I saw and felt it. How could it be false?" But the feeling became so powerful and overwhelming that I could no longer deny it or fight against it. So I tore up the pages I had written, threw myself down on my knees and began to pray, saying, "If it is false, show me how it could be false." And then a voice spoke to my mind and said, *If you had come unto Me, it all would have been different.*

"'I was astounded. I went to church. I read the scriptures often, I prayed pretty regularly, I tried to obey the commandments. "What do you mean, 'Come unto You?'" I wondered. And then into my mind flashed pictures of me wanting to do things my own way, of holding grudges, of not forgiving, of not loving as God had loved us. I had wanted my husband to "pay" for my emotional suffering. I had not let go of the past and had not loved God with all my heart. I loved my own willful self more.

"'I was aghast. I suddenly realized that I was responsible for my own suffering, for if I had really come unto Him, as I outwardly thought I had done, it all *would* have been different. As that horrible truth settled over me, I realized why the pages I had written of my suffering had been false. I had allowed it to happen by not truly coming unto God. That day I repented of not loving God, of not loving my husband, of blaming, of finding fault, of thinking that others were responsible for my misery.

"'I returned home but did not mention to my husband anything of what had transpired. But I gave up blaming, knowing that I was in large part responsible for the state of our relationship. And I tried to come unto God with full purpose of heart. I prayed more earnestly, and listened to His Spirit. I read my scriptures, and tried to come to know Him better.

"'Two months passed, and one morning my husband awoke and turned to me in bed and said, "You know, we find fault too much with each other. I am never going to find fault with my wife again." I was flabbergasted, for he had never admitted he had done anything wrong in our relationship. He did stop finding fault, and he began to compliment me, and show sweet kindness. It was as if an icy glass wall between us had melted away. Almost overnight our relationship became warm and sweet. Three years have passed, and still it continues warmer and happier. We care deeply about one another, and share ideas and thoughts and feelings, something we had not done for the first 16 years of marriage.'"

And then Warner adds: "The Savior seems to say to us: 'Come unto me, and I will give you such assurance and hope and strength that you cannot be taken hostage by anyone who seems to do you harm. I will liberate you into love. And then you will no longer give anyone cause to resent or fear you. Instead, *they* will respond to the love which I have bestowed upon you.'

"Whether it is felt in his breast or in ours, the Savior's love can achieve what force cannot, because where force calls forth counter-force, love calls forth love. In the human image of his divine sacrifice, we too can outlast and conquer vengeance. . . .

". . . . He suffered without taking any offense whatsoever, without becoming mistrustful, without either retaliating or withdrawing or concentrating on himself. . . . Through all [he suffered], there entered into his heart no vindictiveness whatsoever; not even momentarily did his love diminish for any whose pains and sins he bore, including those who in life reviled Him or brutalized His children. . . .

"Rather than resisting evil, he suffered. Rather than compromise, he suffered. Rather than rejecting any of us—though every possible provocation to do so was laid upon him—he suffered. . . . He conquered the forcefulness of force. He defeated all the pressures that push humanity toward enmity and discord. He absorbed the terrible poison of vengeance into himself and metabolized it by his love.

". . . .This love changes everything. . . . No other power calls forth love instead of resistance, changes the heart, and actually makes things better rather than worse. Through his gentle example, by the voice of his Spirit, and in the faces of His children, it awakens us to life. For if we heed its invitation, we are stopped short in our arrogance or self-pity or distraction. We are humbled in our pride or anger or selfishness. Simple humility softens pride and may even redeem it" ("Honest, Simple, Solid, True," *Brigham Young Magazine*, June 1996, 32–39).

Searching My Own Heart

Although I thought before that I had achieved a feeling of peace in regard to my family situation, now peace alluded me. I searched my own heart with more honesty. The phrase from Terry Warner's talk kept returning to me: "If you had come unto me, things would have been very different."

Although at the time I had felt totally justified in my feelings, now my conscience convicted me as I recognized my own self-betrayal through the entire family affair. I knew what I must do.

The following Sunday, a favorite hymn was sung. One of the verses was very appropriate:

> *As now our minds review the past,*
> *We know we must repent;*
> *The way to thee is righteousness—*
> *The way thy life was spent.*
> *Forgiveness is a gift from thee*
> *We seek with pure intent.*

With hands now pledged to do thy work,
We take the sacrament.
        —LEE TOM PERRY

Immediately after services, I received a blessing related to a new assignment. At the end of that short, simple prayer, the man blessed me to be able to make things better with members of my family who had been offended, by showing more love to them. I was shocked. How could he have known what I had been experiencing during the week? Had my husband tipped him off? He had not. It served as one more confirmation that I should proceed with my plan, which was to write to all my siblings and ask their forgiveness.

I had considered myself the innocent victim of my family's cruel ostracism when I was only trying to follow my conscience and do the right thing. Now I looked back to "review the past" with a clearer vision. I recalled the harsh judgments I had formed, the anger in my heart.

I had even told myself I was being Christlike when I didn't respond to their critical letters or defend myself against the false beliefs that were circulating about me. Now I see that I was merely feeling self-righteous, morally superior to them—another face of pride. Truly, I was being a hypocrite, even as I judged and condemned them for being so.

I recognized now that the hard feelings I had harbored were as far from the true gospel of Jesus Christ as they could possibly be. My feelings had been the very antithesis of charity. I had used the way I was being treated as an excuse not to love. I was using their treatment of me to justify my own hard heart.

And all the time that I had struggled, I thought I needed to forgive *them*—when in actuality, *I* was the one who needed to be forgiven.

Even when I felt I *had* forgiven them, with hindsight I see that it was as though I was saying, "I forgive you for *my* having had those un-Christlike feelings toward you." The absurdity of it amazes me now.

At What Price, Pride?

What had I been clinging to? Was pride such a wonderful thing that I didn't want to let go of it? What delightful things would I be deprived of if I let it go? I could think of none. Except, perhaps, the dubious satisfaction of feeling I was "right." But at what price? Could I afford the cost of such an indulgence? ". . . they sell themselves for naught; for, for the reward of their pride and their foolishness they shall reap destruction" (2 Ne. 26:10).

Had pride brought me happiness? Or had it been an obstacle in my professed desire to become more like the Savior, who is meek, submissive, and lowly of heart? What could I possibly lose by choosing to follow Him?

LeGrand Curtis expressed it succinctly: "Truly forgiving one another requires a high commitment to the principles of Christianity. We must keep personal pride under control and put forth an extra measure of love for the person or persons involved."

In surrendering my pride, I would actually be surrendering

to a course that would bring me peace and joy, would open the door to love and draw me closer to God.

A Letter to My Family

In the letter I wrote to my family members, I recounted the events that had led to my change of heart. I was specific in my confessions. For instance, "I had been extremely judgmental, labeling you as being cold and cruel. Now, in facing myself, I had to admit my own guilt. For example, when we sent out birth announcements and invitations to dinner when Merrie Anne was blessed, I knew quite surely that no one would come. The hard truth is that I was (albeit subconsciously, perhaps) actually willing to set up for rejection my own baby daughter in order to prove that I was right about you. Talk about cold and cruel! There may have even been a touch of 'digging a pit for thy neighbor,' as I was inviting or provoking the very behavior that I was condemning you for."

The letter described the realization I had come to of my great need to repent and to be forgiven. "Forgiven for not living the gospel, for following Satan as I harbored resentments and bitterness, for not following the Savior and loving as He loved. For judging others, for feeling myself to be the innocent victim, for nourishing spiritual pride and selfishness in the form of self-pity. For misusing my God-given agency by failing to take responsibility for my own life. For provoking the very behavior I was condemning in others. For not accepting Christ's Atonement and his invitation to bear my burdens for me.

"For all the pain you have experienced because of my lack

in following the Savior, I am truly sorry. I love you all and appreciate the positive things you have added to my life. Even after all this, I can be grateful now, for you have been my best teachers as I have learned from experience and, hopefully, changed and come closer to an awareness of the essence of the true gospel of Jesus Christ and what it means to really follow Him."

CHAPTER SEVENTEEN

It Will Come

*If you are suffering from a bad man's injustice,
forgive him, lest there be two bad men.*
—GILBERT HAY

GORDON B. HINCKLEY offered some comforting words of encouragement. "If there be any who nurture in their hearts the poisonous brew of enmity toward another, I plead with you to ask the Lord for strength to forgive. . . . It may not be easy, and it may not come quickly. But if you will seek it with sincerity and cultivate it, it will come."

A Willing Heart

Perhaps you have felt discouraged, struggling with forgiveness yet not feeling successful in achieving it. Ask yourself, "If I were given the chance to awaken one morning and find my heart full of forgiveness and good will—would I choose to do so? Am I seeking to identify and eliminate negative, judgmental thoughts? Am I making a sincere effort to understand the other person, praying to see him with God's perspective?" If the answer is yes, then you can at least be patient with yourself, recognizing your righteous desires.

The starting point of all change is a sincere heart and a willing mind. We do not need to know *how* to forgive; all we need is to be *willing* to forgive. "For if there be first a willing mind, it is accepted" (2 Cor. 8:12).

If we diligently desire it, the Lord will help us. "Ask, and it shall be given you; seek, and ye shall find; knock, and it shall be opened unto you: For every one that asketh receiveth; and he that seeketh findeth; and to him that knocketh it shall be opened" (Matt. 7:7–8).

So often we seek a change in our condition when what is needed is a change in our attitude. It is one of the happy paradoxes of life that the more ready we are to forgive, the less we are called on to do so.

When we refuse to forgive, we are refusing to allow the light of Christ to have a place in our hearts. No one can be wrong with man and right with God.

A Gallant and Brave Act

Only the brave know how to forgive. A coward never forgave; it is not in his nature. It takes a strong and self-respecting person to have such courage. As one man said, "Nothing is easier than fault finding. No strength, no self-denial, no brains, no character are required to set up in the grumbling business."

It is all love—courageous love and forgiveness—the Master's way of living. Forgiving is the passage to peace and happiness.

Time to Heal

Forgiveness can take time. It deserves the time it needs. But there comes a point at which we must make the decision to stop suffering and start healing. The injury people do to us may seem at the moment to be very great. Yet, just as time heals the wounds of the body, so also does time heal the wounds of the soul. Forgiveness can be viewed as the last step in healing. People who have worked to become forgivers will tell you that it's worth it. Those who haven't may suggest otherwise.

Many years ago, a great heartache came into my life because of the suffering of a loved one. The pain I was sharing and experiencing with her was so intense, so real. I was working then as a secretary at a radio station, and I remember hearing the words of a song that was popular at the time: *"There's got to be a morning after, If we can hold on through the night."* Sometimes, in the pain of the moment, it is   difficult to believe that things will get better, but they do. They do.

After the tempest, calm
After the darkness, light.
And the golden dawn breaks clearly
After the long, long night.

After the rain, the sunshine
After the tears, the laughter.
And when this life is over,
Life eternal follows after.

　　　　　　　　—UNKNOWN

Forgiveness Has Tremendous Power

Forgiveness has tremendous power; it can turn a person's life around. But, because of the principle of free will, it has its limitations. Your forgiveness may never change the person who hurt you. It will not necessarily make others more caring. Your forgiveness may seem miraculous to you, but it may be meaningless to the one you have forgiven. If you can accept this, you can forgive.

As one person observed, "Forgiveness frees us to love again. When we harbor feelings of hurt, anger, and hate in our souls—whether for ourselves or someone else—we choose to allow those negative feelings to canker our souls. We become mired in unhappiness, distress, frustration, and a general malaise of the spirit which prevents us from being able to experience the good feelings which we all need and desire."

A wise man counseled, "Let go. Why do you cling to pain? There is nothing you can do about the wrongs of yesterday. It is not yours to judge. Why hold on to the very thing that keeps you from hope and love?" Forgiveness is an invitation to life. Those who invest energy and emotion into the present will live healthier, happier, and more compassionate lives. They will love their lives.

An 86-year-old woman shared her warm insights, obviously borne of her own experiences. "The joy of complete forgiveness cannot be expressed in words. The feeling of love for the person forgiven is overwhelming. . . . When we truly forgive, all bad thoughts and actions leave our mind. The mind and body rejoice in happiness we cannot feel otherwise. The heavy feeling in our mind leaves, lightness is felt, and we actually feel free of pain. Life seems more wonderful. We feel peace and love."

Forgiving others frees you to let go of your hurt. As the pain leaves you, you realize that any desire to hurt others has gone, too. Forgiveness removes the desire to be spiteful. Forgiveness keeps the channel of love open. It is choosing to allow love to overpower the thing that caused the trouble.

How Do I Know If I Have Truly Forgiven?

Even for relatively small offenses, forgiveness is sometimes an ongoing process requiring consistent, repetitious effort. One woman shared an experience. A young man had stolen all of her family's camping gear—tents, sleeping bags, everything. "I thought I had forgiven him," she said. "But every time I go to get something and remember that it is gone, the feelings return, and I have to go through the forgiveness all over again." She added, "Maybe that's why the scriptures say we need to forgive seventy times seven!"

I have been asked, "How can I tell if I really have forgiven? I *thought* I had forgiven, but now I'm not so sure. How can I know?"

In response to that question, I conducted a little scientific survey—okay, I went to a concert and queried all the people sitting around me before the performance began.

"How do I know if I have forgiven?"

"When I can sincerely wish that person well and not wish for some catastrophe to strike him or think, 'It serves him right,' if some misfortune were to befall him."

"When I no longer feel pain when I think of the experience. By the sense of peace inside me."

"I can tell by how I feel toward that person. Do I still have feelings of revenge? Would I treat him differently because of the incident than if it hadn't happened? It's the way I am with that person. If someone steals from me, I might start locking my door—but how I treat the *person* shows that I have forgiven him."

"I know I've forgiven when I can think about the incident or think of that person and can see that person as a child of God instead of in a negative way."

"When the other person and I can feel comfortable together and not think about the incident that caused the harmful feelings."

"When I don't feel any hatred toward them anymore. When I don't bring it up again; I don't recall it, even in my own mind."

"When I no longer feel pain. When I no longer dwell on it in my thoughts. When I no longer feel a need to talk to other people about it. When I'm ready to forget it and go on with my life."

"When I can look them in the eye and be glad that they are around me—when I don't remember what they did."

"Because I don't worry about it anymore. It doesn't bother me anymore."

"I have forgotten—most of the time. When it no longer innervates me. It is past; there is nothing lingering."

"I know I'd forgiven because I would have forgotten it and would love them again."

I found these responses rather interesting in that they seemed quite similar. We know we've forgiven by the feelings that *we* have inside. Forgiveness is not about *them*; it is about *us*. No one mentioned a requirement that the offending person has expressed his sorrow or has begged for our forgiveness. The responsibility to forgive rests with us, not in their asking for it. It is our own peace that depends upon it.

I've found a little remedy to ease the life we live,
And make each day a happier one—
It is the word, "Forgive."

So often little things, if given up at once,
Would not amount to anything.
'Tis when we hold them up to view,
And brood and sulk and fret,
They greater grow before our eyes.
'Twas better to forget.

So when at night you seek your bed,
Ere yet your eyelids close,
Lay all your problems, doubts, and fears,
Before the One who knows.

And await the verdict of the One
Who knows just why you live,

And hear the blessed words of peace:
"Forgive, as I forgive."
—UNKNOWN

A Feeling of Connectedness

Forgiveness comes more easily when we feel connected with God's other children. Viewing ourselves and others as one, as part of a whole, will give us an entirely different perspective on forgiveness. Perhaps this is what at-one-ment means.

One woman stated, "To participate in the atonement, we have to *be one with others,* and we can't achieve this if there is emotional distance created by not forgiving others."

When a blanket was stolen from the car of one man, he expressed sorrow—not for his loss, but for the fact that he had not known someone needed it. "I would have *given* it to him," he said.

One person defined forgiveness as being "when we channel our thoughts and feelings so that *we look at the other person as being ourself,* knowing that we also have weaknesses and have also provided hurtful situations for others that we would hope to be forgiven for."

Another agreed. "It is a realization of the imperfection of humanity and making allowances for that imperfection, knowing we *all* suffer from the same malady."

Another stated, "Forgiveness is the willingness to love someone no matter what they do. If you can't forgive, you can't love, since *everyone* makes mistakes."

Still another said, "Forgiveness is the ability to think beyond one's own needs to another person's feelings, and clear the other person of feeling guilt or sadness over wrong committed, intentionally or not."

When we feel connected to all mankind, realizing that we are all part of God's family, we know that either we suffer together, or we rejoice together. One cannot help or hurt another without helping or hurting himself, because we are all part of a whole. Reaching out and giving become natural.

It is impossible to create any bitterness or hatred toward others when your primary objective is to be a giving human being. Giving and forgiving come almost automatically when you no longer feel separate, looking out for yourself first, focusing on getting. It is a paradox that the less you are obsessed with getting and the more willing you are to reach out to others and give, the more you seem to get.

Forgiveness begins when we are able to look upon the wrongdoer as we look upon ourselves. So often, we perceive ourselves and others as separate, causing us to judge unfairly. We may be prone, then, to judge others by their actions and ourselves by our intentions.

As one person stated, "We upset the balance or equality of mankind when we put ourselves above another and cannot grant forgiveness. We cannot find this balance in our lives unless we treat others as equals and let go of self-righteousness."

We cannot truly forgive from a position of superiority, what David Augsburger terms "one-up forgiveness." It is as though we are saying: "I have examined, weighed, judged you and your behavior and found you sorely lacking in qualities that are worthy of my respect. I have these qualities at this point in time, but you do not. I humbly recognize my superior moral strength and your weakness. I forgive you your trespasses. We will henceforth have a relationship based on the recognition of my benevolence in the hour of your neediness, my generosity in the face of your guilt. You will find some suitable way to be dutifully grateful from this day forward."

True forgiveness flows from real love, unconditional love, a genuine concern for another. It requires a pure heart and integrity of soul as we acknowledge our connectedness with each other and our equality and oneness before God.

Our Great Task

A wise man stated, "We are here on this earth to learn two things: how to repent and how to forgive."

Learning to forgive is one of the most important things you will ever do. If you feel discouraged that you have had some difficulty, at least be assured that the struggle will be worth it. A teacher once said, "The holiest of all spots on earth is where an ancient hatred has become a present love."

I can assure you that if you are sincere in your desire, you *can* succeed in achieving a forgiving heart. "If any man has a quarrel against any: even as Christ forgave you, *so also do ye*" (Col. 3:13; emphasis added). If it were not possible to forgive, God would not have commanded it. It will come.

Our purpose is to one day return to live with our Creator, where love is complete and pure. Our task here is to prepare ourselves by learning to love others unconditionally. We do this best through forgiveness.

Certainly, forgiveness is the healing gift we give ourselves. But more accurately, it is a gift from the Master, the way to eternal life. *He* is the One who offers the gift; *we* must decide whether or not we will receive it.

"May God grant unto you that your burdens may be light, through the joy of his Son. And even all this ye can do, *if ye will*" (Alma 33:23).

Epilogue

I T HAS BEEN five years since the trouble in my family began. No—the trouble could not have begun five years ago, for, in truth, "circumstances do not make the man—they only reveal him to himself." I suspect the problem may have been with us always. The unfortunate situation that divided my family only crystallized and revealed what was already the state of our hearts.

It was not pleasant for me to face the reality of what lay in my *own* heart. That new awareness, painful as it was to acknowledge, brought me, nine months ago, to write the letter to my seven siblings in which I confessed my need for repentance and asked their forgiveness.

There was no immediate or direct response to the letter. It would have been unrealistic of me to have hoped for any—the chasm was too wide, the abyss too deep. Moreover, an expectation of seeing such results would have been an indication that I had written the letter for the wrong reason—as a means of manipulating others to obtain a desired result. That was not my intent; it was my *own* heart that had changed.

Later, I happened upon the following scripture: "If they have not charity it mattereth not unto thee, thou hast been faithful; wherefore, thy garments shall be made clean. And because thou hast seen thy weakness thou shalt be made strong" (Ether 12:36–37).

For the most part, the official ostracism continues. This, despite our 80-year-old mother's sorrow and increasing distress as, over time, she has witnessed the pride and prejudice pervading hearts, preventing reconciliation.

Recently, however, we have experienced minor miracles, small indications that hearts might be softening. Like the warm reception by a brother and his family when my husband and I traveled to another state and spent a day with my mother this spring. More recently, the visit of a brother and his family—one who just two months previously had chosen not to see me during that same trip. Another brother and his wife joining us at our table at a cousin's wedding reception. The chance meeting in a grocery store with the most offended brother. There was a time when I would have quickly turned and headed the opposite direction, but now my reaction upon seeing him was to say, "My brother!" and to give him a hug, to which he responded in a positive way, thankfully.

A delightful evening was spent with yet another brother who came alone to make a request for photographs to be included in an upcoming issue of the family newsletter—although, he said almost apologetically, I still would not be receiving a copy of the newsletter nor be invited to contribute in any way other than the photos. During our visit, he divulged that, upon receiving my letter, his first inclination had been to immediately contact me and express his love — although he apparently resisted the impulse.

I have had to reconcile myself to the fact that some things I may never comprehend. I have given up trying to make sense of the situation and have had to give it to God to sort out. As someone said, "It has taken me a long time to understand that I don't have to understand everything."

Months after writing my letter of apology, I received a beautiful card from my only sister in which she wrote, "Thank you for the letter. I know that you are trying to do what's right. Please know that I love you and pray for the time that we can be of one accord as a family.

"I think about you often, and pray for you, and for all our loved ones. We all have need of repentance — and forgiveness."

In a subsequent letter, she disclosed the reason that she had been moved to write me: "It was because of a dream I had one day as I napped. I dreamed that Mom and you and I were all together again, here in my living room. And it was just like old times. And as I woke up, the realization hit me that it may never happen again. I awoke just sobbing."

We have since shared a visit — our mother, my sister, and me. Only, because of my two broken legs, it was in the confines of my bedroom rather than her living room!

While the situation in my family still causes me a degree of sadness, it no longer occupies center stage in my life and my thoughts. Perhaps forgiving *is* forgetting. I no longer feel a need or desire to discuss the circumstances with others; those issues no longer seem significant. The offenses and exclusions might continue, but I pay them little heed. No longer do I feel the pain I previously felt so intensely. Time *does* heal. There are so many happy people and plans and projects in my life! I choose to focus upon my blessings in the present rather than dwelling on the pain of the past. I don't live there anymore.

I am grateful for the precious truths I have learned through this experience. At the same time, I recognize that each of us is on his own journey. Life *will* give us opportunities to learn— sometimes willingly, sometimes not. It is not my place to judge another's progress in his journey; God has asked us to leave judgment to Him. What a relief to finally understand that.

In the meantime, I still have much to learn! I have gained a stronger conviction of the vital need for unconditional love. I believe now that we are all meant to be loving creatures; it is our divine nature. It is when we *resist* the natural, God-given inclination to love that we experience inner conflict and a lack of peace.

But that is the topic of another book. Perhaps it will be titled, *You Don't Deserve My Unconditional Love,* or *Confessions of a Modern-day Pharisee.* Until then, I wish you blessings on your journey. . . .

Sources

Brinkley, Dannion, *Saved by the Light* (Rockland: Wheeler Publishing, 1994)

Cramer, Steven, *The Worth of a Soul* (Orem: Randall Book, 1983)

Cramer, Steven, *In the Arms of His Love* (American Fork: Covenant Communications, 1991)

Dyer, Wayne, *You'll See It When You Believe It* (Newark: Avon Books)

Eadie, Betty J., *The Awakening Heart* (New York: Pocket Books, 1996)

Flaherty, Sandra M., *Women, Why Do You Weep? Spirituality for Survivors of Childhood Sexual Abuse* (Mahwah: Paulist Press, 1992)

Fox, Emmet, *The Sermon on the Mount: The Key to Success in Life* (New York: Harper-Collins Publishers, 1938)

Furey, Robert J., *The Joy of Kindness* (New York: Crossroad Publishing, 1993)

Gayton, Richard, *The Forgiving Place, "Choosing Peace After Violent Trauma"* (Waco: WRS Publishing, 1995)

Jaramillo, Cato, *Too Stubborn to Die* (Carson City: Goldleaf Press, 1995)

Newell, Lloyd D., *The Divine Connection* (Salt Lake City: Deseret Book Company, 1992)

ten Boom, Corrie, *The Hiding Place* (Ada: Flemming H. Revell Co., 1996)

Ulrich, Wendy, *Spiritual Recovery,* "When Forgiveness Flounders: For Victims of Serious Sin"

Warner, C. Terry, *Bonds of Anguish, Bonds of Love* (Unpublished book manuscript available at Kimball Tower Copy Center, BYU, Provo, Utah)

Washington, Booker T., *Up from Slavery* (Nineola: Dover Publications, Inc., 1995)

Scripture verses from *The Old Testament* and *The New Testament*, King James Version; *The Doctrine and Covenants* (D&C); *The Book of Mormon, Another Testament of Jesus Christ* (2 Nephi, [2 Ne.] Alma, Ether, Mormon [Morm.] Helaman [Hel.] and Moroni [Moro.]); and *The Pearl of Great Price* (Moses); published by the Church of Jesus Christ of Latter-day Saints, Salt Lake City, Utah, U.S.A.

Material originally published in the *Ensign* magazine, The Church of Jesus Christ of Latter-day Saints, is reprinted by permission.

About the Author

CHERYL CARSON is a popular speaker and writer, having authored several books, booklets, and numerous articles. She has lectured at Brigham Young University Campus Education Week, Best of Especially for Youth, and at hundreds of youth conferences and workshops at BYU and in 12 states. In addition to the subjects of forgiveness and of unconditional love, Cheryl writes and speaks on a variety of subjects including: *The Anguish—and Adventure—of Adversity; With Parents Kind and Dear: A Gentler, More Christlike Approach to Raising Children; The Me I See Is the Me I'll Be; and Chastity—Now and Forever.* She has also been a frequent guest on a local radio talk show for a number of years.

Committed to her church, Cheryl has served as president of youth and children's organizations and in many other leadership capacities.

She is the mother of four adopted children, five stepchildren and two "homemade" babies. Cheryl and her husband, Micheal, live in Provo, Utah, with a fluctuating number of children.

Cheryl Carson
256 North 2370 West
Provo, Utah 84601
(801)374-5686